on smaller
dogs and
larger life
questions

on smaller dogs and larger life questions

KATE FIGES

virago

VIRAGO

First published in Great Britain in 2018 by Virago Press

1 3 5 7 9 10 8 6 4 2

A CIP catalogue record for this book
is available from the British Library.

ISBN 978-0-349-01102-8

Typeset in Plantin by M Rules
Printed and bound in Great Britain by
Clays Ltd, St Ives plc

Papers used by Virago are from well-managed forests
and other responsible sources.

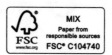

MIX
Paper from
responsible sources
FSC
www.fsc.org   FSC® C104740

Virago Press
An imprint of
Little, Brown Book Group
Carmelite House
50 Victoria Embankment
London EC4Y 0DZ

An Hachette UK Company
www.hachette.co.uk

www.virago.co.uk

For my family
With all my love

That which your hands
Have touched
Has since perished
Slowly the fire of life
Turns all that lives to black dust
However, all that your heart
Has touched
And cherished
Has survived. Only love
Lives longer than us.

Olga Chugai (1944–2015)
Translated by Philip Nikolayev

contents

zeus

Zeus is a miniature wire-haired dachshund, a survivor from a litter of six. His mother had a difficult birth and couldn't look after her babies. So the breeder stepped in as surrogate, feeding the three remaining puppies with a pipette every hour and cuddling them through the first weeks of life to keep them warm. Zeus was her miracle, she said as the only surviving male made straight for us at our first meeting, demanding to be picked up. How could we not be smitten and feel the need to bring this tiny bundle of fluff with seductive eyes into our family?

Within days the four of us – my two daughters, my husband and me – were exchanging emails with silly suggestions for names – Basil, Nigel, Ebucadnezer. We bought him an expensive blue basket to sleep in, as well as toys, chews, poo bags, training mats to pee on, a collar and a lead. We had his home phone number engraved on a disc to hang from his collar so that we would never lose him. And when we triumphantly brought him home, just eighteen months after our beloved first dachshund had died, his arrival blasted apart my life.

The pressure for a new dog had been quiet but persistent. I knew that having a puppy to hug and care for would fill a different hole in each of our lives. I knew too that a dog would reunite the four adult wings of our family by giving us a project to share, some little being to care for and love passionately. And so it was proving. We emailed each other witty captions attached to photographs – his first trip to the park, encounters with ducks and pigeons, endearing attempts at cocking his leg against a tree like a big dog before falling over, looking like a lost orphan sitting by himself on a bench at Dalston station. It was heartwarming to see how just holding this little puppy brought such joy and comfort to my daughters, who were going through all the big things that haunt young women in their twenties. Zeus was like a living teddy bear. He lolled about in their arms and loved nothing more than to be cosseted like a baby. He gave us all something to talk about and play with.

When you have small children, dogs slide easily into the family groove. They play together and are good for each other. You go to the park to get the kids running around in the fresh air, so the dog comes along too. Home is inevitably messy, with half-eaten yoghurts and bananas, piles of toys and clothes waiting to be put away or into the washing machine, and with small children there is already so much mud on the carpet and poo to deal with that a little more passes unnoticed. A dog is a healthy distraction *from* the children. When you feel underappreciated, or the object of deep loathing from a teenager because you have denied them some unalienable right like going to a party a hundred miles from home without a means of getting back on a school night, the dog still loves you unconditionally. He, at least, is always pleased to see you and thanks you with a wagging tail for that choccy droppie treat.

Then the children grow up – and away. The ageing parents, for many – including me – are also, sadly, gone. You begin to get used to being free from the anxieties of caring for more vulnerable and dependent beings. You have time to think about what you might want from each day rather than putting the wants and needs of others first. You don't have to go to the park unless you want to. You will probably never achieve half of what you imagine you might, but it's a liberating thought to be able to have all the same. Suddenly all that freedom, all that new sense of being able to be truly selfish for the first time in my life, vanished with the arrival of just one small puppy.

Suddenly, I was housebound again and like a new mother, filled with anxiety about the dog: whether he was chewing through an electric wire, or about to pee on the floor. As a freelancer based at home, I became the one who had to monitor his welfare, care for his needs and stay with him while the others got on with the rest of their lives, just as they had always done. If I needed to go out I had to shut this squealing puppy into his crate and then worried about whether he was all right until I got back.

Post-Canine Acquisition threw me back to the trapped feelings of powerlessness and inadequacy I felt after the birth of my first baby nearly thirty years ago. My needs suddenly succumbed to those of the puppy. The exhaustion in those first few weeks, as he learned to sleep through the night, the constant clearing up of his mess on our new carpet and trying not to scold him because that isn't the way you're supposed to do it any more, the hours spent standing in the freezing cold of our small patio garden, waiting for him to pee so that I could praise him for doing it in the right place, were more tiring than I ever remembered with our first dog. It had all happened such a long time ago. And though my husband helped, of course, we were both much older now. With less energy.

Somehow this responsibility for a small, fragile living being tore open a deep wound in me. I felt oversensitive, once again tender inside, reminding me of the years of close mothering. I had forgotten how it felt to have a constant and acute anxiety about the welfare of those who are vulnerable and in your care, which in turn provokes feelings of inadequacy and resentment even because you cannot possibly protect them from every chance horror in life. The great relief of having grown-up daughters is that

I don't know what they get up to from one day to the next, so I just can't worry about the minutiae and daily dangers.

My anxiety over Zeus when he got ill with gastroenteritis just six weeks after his arrival was so acute that I wondered at one point if I might be about to have a stroke. Did I want him to live or die? Of course I hoped this small bundle of joy would survive. Didn't I? We had already invested so much in him. But there was also a sneaky, guilty chink of light, a beckoning back to the freedom I had lost.

After four good nights' sleep without Zeus we brought him home. And then suddenly it all got too much. I started crying and couldn't stop, just like I used to when I was a child, almost every night into my pillow as I imagined my father coming back to rescue me and take me off to a happier place. I cried so easily then. My father told me I had to toughen up and be less sensitive. As if that was easy, like turning off a tap.

This new mid-life crisis over the dog and exhaustion and caring seemed to provoke similar tears, resonating with that vulnerable little girl. Approaching sixty, with the confinement of the dog, I was beginning to feel just as unseen and insignificant as I had done as a child; I felt again that somehow my needs didn't seem to matter as much as everybody else's. I was astonished and overwhelmed by the swelling grief and sadness that revealed a deep, buried vulnerability. And it seemed that all it took was one small puppy.

Ashamed of my inability to cope with an animal so small that I could strangle it with just one hand, I feigned happiness. But alone the tears tumbled onto the little creature in my lap who chewed at my fingers and then clambered up onto my chest to lick my cheeks dry. I became almost willingly isolated and trapped by this dog.

I could no longer hide the fact that I had begun to shirk company, to slob around in old clothes. My daughters and my husband, Christoph, told me I was depressed, that I needed therapy. My misery was pushing them away. But it's just the dog, I said. This bloody dog. I am drained dry. There is nothing left to give. They didn't believe me.

Why had I agreed to the puppy? My mother's default position to any request was usually negative, and when my daughters were small I could hear her in my head as 'No' tumbled out of my mouth at the most benign request, such as 'Can I have a banana?' Is that why I said yes now? Or was it because I sensed a vacuum left by children growing up and moving away? Did I actually need something that needed me for total care? It is always easier to slip into the same, well-trodden ways rather than to branch out bravely and take on something new. Or maybe I hadn't said no because I wanted to make my loved ones happy. I have always wanted to be the kind of mother I felt mine never was: someone who always put her family first. But, I now mused, maybe what that means is giving too much and then resenting it. Was saying yes a mistake?

I found it hard to say a clear no or yes as a child. 'I don't mind' was my usual timid answer. I exasperated my father in a fish restaurant with sawdust on the floor in Baker Street, a place where he liked to go when he had us for the day so that he could flirt with the waitresses and smoke heavily over endless cups of black coffee, because I couldn't choose between chocolate or vanilla ice cream. 'Choose!' he said, almost yelling. 'Which one do you want the most?' But I didn't know. Having a definite opinion on anything felt risky.

My parents hated each other. Anything I said could exacerbate their fury and so I believed that if I faded into the background then maybe all of their rows would stop. I had learned that what I really wanted didn't matter anyway. I had wanted my father to stay but nobody had asked me and he left.

Meanwhile, whatever I thought and felt, Zeus grew stronger, slept through the night and became more or less house-trained. The emotional crisis he had provoked thankfully seemed to be subsiding. I arranged puppy-sitters and dog-walkers. Life was getting back on track.

But then came the diagnosis.

My existential crisis had not been provoked by the arrival of a puppy.

I was seriously ill.

*

For a while I had ignored mild muscle aches around my ribs and back. When they turned into sharp pains I went to the doctor. Test upon test, and each seemed to reveal more bad news. It could be my heart. An X-ray showed a shadow on my lung. A scan showed fractured ribs and multiple lytic lesions: holes in the bones indicating myeloma – bone-marrow cancer. Then, a bone-marrow biopsy revealed a very different story: a breast cancer primary.

I had had regular mammograms, examined my breasts for lumps and assumed that the dull shoulder ache and occasional itching beneath my left breast was just what happens when you sit hunched over a laptop for hours or play too much tennis. And, like many women, I had no idea that some breast cancers are so small they cannot be seen in a mammogram. But it says so in the small print of the letter, below the good news that your breasts are clear.

How fitting that it should be breast, that symbol of love and maternal feeding, that became the target of cancerous activity, and not the bowel or the liver. Unsurprisingly, all my anxieties about the dog drained away.

I have triple negative breast cancer, the most aggressive kind, 'treatable but not curable'.

No wonder I couldn't cope.

Suddenly we were shunted sideways into a parallel universe, on to Planet Cancer, where only it and whatever the next test showed mattered. With just one snap of the fingers I had turned from someone who rarely took a painkiller, someone who was fit and actively thrusting her way through the world, to a cancer patient, sucked into the orbit of oncologists, uncertainty and the likelihood of strong, highly toxic medication.

It took just four weeks to go from sharp pains in my ribs to this staggering diagnosis. Four weeks of feeling suspended in mid-air, knowing that the outcome wasn't going to be good but clinging to the possibility that it could be otherwise. It was osteoporosis, surely. The tests were wrong. There were irrational moments of slim hope between results. 'Good news: I have unusual blood,' I tell a friend on the phone as I stroll down from the doctor's triumphantly. 'I'm one of the less than 1 per cent of people for whom myeloma doesn't show up in the blood. I have special blood. Yay!' When a PET-CT scan told us that I didn't have primaries elsewhere, indicating once again that this was likely to be myeloma, a disease I'd never heard of before, this seemed like profoundly good news, and again something to celebrate.

When the bone-marrow biopsy confirmed that this was breast cancer that had moved into the bone, I spent an agonising ninety minutes waiting to see the breast specialist at the end of his patient list. I paced the waiting room trying to breathe deeply. I looked out of the window at the sky and tried to calm myself. I was up in a helicopter looking down, telling myself that soon this nightmare of uncertainty would be over. It was just one small speck of difficulty in a life full of so many more ups than downs.

When I finally got to see the oncologist he was charming, charismatic and good-looking, which helped. But he didn't mince his words. 'People usually ask me if this is terminal . . . ' Terminal? That thought had never occurred to me. 'But that's only the case if I can't treat you, and there are treatments which will help us beat this back and keep it in your bones. The good news is that you won't need surgery and it isn't in your vital organs.' Good news. 'But you have to get on top of this pain, because pain zaps energy and positivity and you are going to need both to get through this.' Great. Give me morphine. We staggered home.

It was too big a concept to grasp, too big a change to our happy, healthy, stable lives. This wasn't in the plan, the future we had imagined for ourselves, travelling and revelling in the post-child-raising years, growing old together slowly. The girls looked devastated and started googling and talking in terms of 'stages'. What? Don't even go there. I don't want to know. I'm not dead yet and don't plan to be any time soon and you certainly cannot start divvying up my clothes.

This is the great fear of mid-life suddenly made real. We pretend that we're still young. We kid ourselves that we have all the time in the world to relax and do all the things we want when we eventually retire. Like most people, I hadn't thought much about death or dying, other than in the most basic intellectual terms, until that great fickle finger of fate pointed down from the heavens at me and only me and said 'You're done for. Unimportant. Surplus to requirements.' My overwhelming feeling was, and still is, one of sadness that I might not be there for Stoph and the girls. It was what my family rather than what I might lose which upset me the most. I have failed them by getting this ill.

Having cancer makes me feel like I have been taken over by an alien being. Oddly, it's rather like being pregnant: I am harbouring something with a life force of its own, feeding off my energy so that it can grow. It is separate, yet a part of me. It makes me feel very, very tired and it is hard to move around because of the pain. Having a baby is almost always entirely positive, a fresh life and new beginnings. But with this there is only the destructive, ugly, pernicious haunt of endings.

There are other similarities to pregnancy and motherhood. It's such a seismic life change that your sense of self is utterly transformed, and in this case, trashed. You can never go back to being the person you once were, before the diagnosis. There are the extreme mood swings from the depths of despair to the sheer joy of being alive, just as I felt with small children. There are the sleepless nights because of the anxiety. I can only sleep on my back, not my sides, because of the cracked ribs, as three pathological fractures from the cancer chomp away at my bones. With mothering, plans change at a moment's notice when a child is ill. Now plans change because I feel too sick or tired from the treatment; my days are punctuated by juicing and the taking of supplements, regulated the way it used to be with baby feeds, bath-time, stories and bed.

Losing control isn't easy for someone with a chaotic, insecure childhood. I need to know that I am doing everything possible to make sure that nothing threatening happens. Only it just has. This will be the hardest aspect of living on Planet Cancer: giving in to the new life I now have to lead.

Within days of the diagnosis, the pain in my ribs and back increased dramatically. Muscle spasms grabbed at my torso, spasms so acute they reminded me again of childbirth. I couldn't walk much or climb the stairs. Only baths and hot-water bottles helped. I gobbled painkillers, and with no light at the end of the tunnel, no certainty that this agony would ever end, I began to wonder whether it really wouldn't be better just to die now, particularly as I couldn't even get comfort from the most basic human comfort – hugs. I began to feel terrified of anyone coming close in case they should hurt me. I was trapped inside another unreachable bubble.

Cancer can feel isolating. There's still a stigma attached to the disease even though so many people get it. You no longer inhabit the same terrain as your cancer-free friends and that's a very lonely feeling. Surprisingly, some of my oldest friends avoid me completely; others seem to see only the illness not me, eyes lowered, unable to find the right words to say, as if I am dead already. This is their fear talking, of their own mortality rather than their fears for me. When their faces crumple with sympathy and their eyes fill with tears, I want to say get a grip. I am the one who might be dying, not you. Yet.

Year One on Planet Cancer requires monumental amounts of self-care – hard for most women, who have a habit of looking after others before themselves. And that's a weird one, which is going to take some getting used to. As is the overwhelming sense of love from those closest to me.

The phone started to ring, and ring. It's Christoph who takes the calls. I hear the tiredness in his voice, with every emotion held back as he spells out the details of the past day or week with journalistic accuracy. He has been a stalwart, loving presence. There was only one outburst of carer's resentment, with a moan of 'What do you want *now?*' He never likes to leave my side. 'We are in this together,' he says as he squeezes my hand in the waiting room before yet another doctor's appointment. He carries a notebook with him and writes down everything they say, a second pair of ears. But I can sense his feelings of inadequacy at not being able to ease my agony as he helps me into yet another hot bath or up to bed. I see the deep crevices of anxiety etched into his forehead as I moan with pain. I can sense that he believes me to be in a bad way.

With the grace and generosity of a gentleman he insists I do not waste an ounce of unnecessary energy on chores or pointless tasks, and instead invest everything in getting better. He fusses around me, making sure I have taken my painkillers and that water is always within reach. He has moved his office into mine so that he can make me green tea or fill a hot-water bottle between emails. He has learned how to cook more than just a fish pie, goes out shopping regularly for food and now separates the whites from the coloureds before loading them into the washing machine. All of this and more I used to do for him and our daughters, but cannot any more, so weak am I that even bending down is painfully impossible.

Growing up with an absent, unreliable father made it difficult for me to trust men, and for the first ten years of our marriage I used to ask regularly, 'You're not going to leave me, are you?' Now, after nearly three decades of the most warm and wonderful marriage, when I am at my most vulnerable and needy, I know that he is there. He can make me laugh at the darkest times and I cannot believe how lucky I am. Knowing that women are likely to be queuing up on the doorstep with casseroles, should I die soon, is enough to keep me alive. He is with me and I intend to keep it that way.

I see how anxious and frightened my daughters are, and yet they rise to the challenge of caring for me with a purity of love that takes me by surprise; it flows without the slightest hint of resentment. They shop for healthy foods and cook. They clear up the mess, massage my feet, tie my shoelaces and think of nice things to do to cheer me up. They fill me up with their love. When I was younger I did the right things as a dutiful daughter, shopping for my mother when she was ill, visiting regularly, telephoning daily and involving her in my family life, but that never seemed to be enough. She wanted more and the result was that we both felt abandoned and resentful. But love is earned, not owed out of a sense of duty. And all the love I have given my two is pouring back into me, refilling the place where giving comes from.

My dear brother calls and texts often, and visits every Tuesday with 'meals on wheels'. He has bought a special bag so that he can transport the dishes. He wants to talk about the diagnosis, how I am feeling, over and over again as slowly the truth drips in that his older sister might not be there for him much longer. He wants to buy me things, and I know he would stop at nothing if I said it would make my life easier. I love him all the more for it. The little brother I adore and have spent my life looking out for, through our parents' divorce and all the shit that life can throw, now wants to look after me.

Neighbours check in on us daily to see if we need anything. I see more of many of my friends than I ever used to when I was healthy. They call often. They come round with lunch, supper and presents. We talk openly about the diagnosis and what it might mean. They offer comfort when I cry and encourage me to be positive, to look after myself, to believe in a future. When I lie against her gift – a cashmere-covered two-foot-long hot-water bottle to soothe the aches in my back – I think of my dear friend Flora. When I walk slowly to the park, for those all-important thirty minutes of gentle exercise, wrapping Heti's scarf around my neck and squirting Bee's perfume, the one she wears herself, about my clothes, I take them with me too. Lying back on the giant cushion knitted for me by Fanny, beneath the beautiful checked throw sent by Helen, I smile. When I have my daily oolong tea, my 'Lee-tea', I think of the dear man who sent me a Jing glass tea set and the most delicious Li Shan oolong tea. Cassia is there when I massage glowing cream into my face or tip delicious-smelling bath salts under hot running water. And when nobody comes to see me I look at the flowers that arrive almost daily. New friends have come into my life too, bringing DVDs, soap and sage advice. So many people have had cancer that they understand and want to bring support. More than that, these are people I really like. People I wish I had got to know years ago.

It feels incongruous with the patterns of the past, where I felt I had to give more to others than I took from them to justify myself and our friendships. Now others are giving everything they can to me. In spades. I never knew that I was this loved, that I could be *this* loved. I am being held high in the arms of a warm embrace from a wide community of friends and family and I know this will help to heal me. What getting Zeus and then cancer has revealed is that I am drained of energy and even the ability to love. Now, in this pit of despair, I might finally be learning how to let others love and care for me. Kindness and caring for others – whether they are human beings or dogs – epitomises the best of who we are.

But it's shit. No doubt about it. Still, it is the first genuinely bad thing that has happened to us in nearly thirty years, as I tell my daughters repeatedly. They are not children any more and it is me, not them, mercifully, who is this ill. I have no choice but to find ways to change and adapt to this new state of 'normality'. I may be ill and my daily life may be compromised, but there is some consolation in an emerging awareness and the beginnings of an acceptance of how short life can be.

I look out of the car window as Christoph drives me to doctor's appointments, scans and treatment, at the crowds of people, hurrying around central London, far more active than I can be but with such tension etched into their furrowed brows. It could be you next, I think as I watch a woman walking, with difficulty, in high heels through the entrance to a Tube station, or you, sir, in your smart, dark suit, running across the road in front of us. For nearly one in two are likely to be diagnosed with cancer at some point in their lives. Everyone lives with the uncertainty of will it be me? I live knowing that it is me. And with that knowledge I have no choice but to surrender to what matters most – my family, friends and loving others while I can.

*

Zeus is now eighteen months old and I love him more and more each day. He struts around our basement like he owns the place, a stroppy teenager pushing back the boundaries of discipline or reverting to puppydom as he leaps like a March hare upon an empty plastic water bottle. He is a central and crucial part of our lives. His unmitigated, innocent enthusiasm for life is infectious. He melts my heart. He allows us to revel in the escapist joy of play, wrestling with ropes or throwing balls for him to retrieve.

Christoph takes him for a walk each morning and not just for the exercise; it gets him out and away from me. The girls look after Zeus whenever they can, taking him to work in a bookshop where he has no doubt helped to increase sales, and to bars and cafés where he is the star of the show. And when I am alone with him, he looks at me tenderly as if to say 'Are you OK?' before climbing carefully onto my lap. Or he presses his paw delicately on my foot when I am sitting at the kitchen table, just to say 'Hi, I'm here . . . pick me up if you can.'

I wonder now whether my breakdown with his arrival was my body trying to tell me that I was ill. Ironically, the one thing that I really resented about having a puppy was having to be home most of the time. And yet now that I am confined to the house he has become one of my greatest comforts. We lie together on the sofa and argue over who has more of a right to the hot-water bottle. He is innocent and happy, a benign being to cuddle and curl up with, unless I fart loudly – chemo plays havoc with the digestion. Then he jumps off the sofa, revolted by the smell, and throws a dirty look at me as he heads for his basket.

A dog's life flies by so much faster than ours. Puppies turn from being adolescent at the age of one to grumpy old men in not much more than a decade. We will watch time speed up for Zeus just as it does for me now. There is nothing like a cancer diagnosis when it comes to shining a bright light on the blinding, clichéd truism that life is far, far too short. You can never quite believe that when you think you have a whole lifetime of empty space ahead of you to fill. I try to capture the sounds, smells, light and miracle of being alive. We are one now, Zeus and I, on much the same continuum. And it is anybody's guess as to who will have to be put down first.

tennis

I always knew that the day would come when I wouldn't be able to play tennis any more, I just didn't think it would be so soon. But that's the thing with cancer. You're fine, breezing along, feeling on top of your game, with a devilish cross-court backhand, and then BANG! Breast cancer that has gone into the bone.

The pains had started after a particularly competitive game with friends one Sunday morning. Christoph and I were losing badly at mixed doubles – 0–3 down. Middle age means that we only ever have enough energy for one set before the need for lunch and a bottle of wine takes over. So, a poor loser, I decided to dig deep, serving with venom and fathoming levels of competitiveness I can only remember feeling once before, in sprint races in PE, when there was a girl I hated running in the lane beside me. I won then. And that Sunday we beat our opponents 6–4.

For the next few days my ribs were sore, my shoulders ached from serving, but it was worth it, for that glint of glory from a decisive comeback.

Playing tennis liberates all those unseemly-for-a-girl emotions. You can get nasty and even hit balls at people's heads. You're expected to want to win and allowed to whoop with guilt-free joy when you score a particularly good point; you can shout and vent your frustration when you miss an easy shot. You can do it all, provided you abide by the rules of the game and apologise when the ball hits the net before dropping pleasingly down onto their side of the court. The etiquette then is clear. You hold up your racket face, even though everybody knows you're not really sorry at all, but thrilled at the prospect of a serendipitous point. And then you graciously shake hands with your opponents at the end.

Over the past ten years I have walked to the park in all weathers, eager to play and to work on my technique with friends found through a shared love of the game. This was for me a personal pleasure entirely devoid of anything useful or productive; happiness comes when you can lose yourself in something for no particular purpose. The rest of the world and all my problems slipped away as I focused on nothing but the ball. What could matter more in that moment as it came hurtling towards me other than how to hit it? Forehand or backhand? Run in to volley or leave it for your partner? Snap decisions as you aim, hit and pray that it lands in that sweet spot within the white lines and the point is yours.

I loved the softness of the ball in my hand as I tossed it high into the air to serve: bright yellow against a blue and white sky. I loved the smell of it, a tinge of plastic merged with a hint of sweaty palms and the decay of falling leaves. I loved the way the bounce was different in hot or cold weather and I loved that thwack as the ball flew from plumb in the middle of my racket. I loved the feel of the handle swaddled in a soft, squishy grip as I squeezed it in the palm of my hand just before hitting the ball. I loved the way my pulse quickened with excitement and I loved the smell of my sunburned skin, of dried sweat, as the weeks of summer passed.

Tennis changed my life. If I couldn't play for a week I felt low and sluggish. I missed it. Tennis got me out to notice the changing colours of the trees, the volatility of weather. The physicality of it, the way my muscles ached after a good morning's play, the growing respect I found for the capability of my legs, the way it made me fitter and empowered me as I slowly improved at something I was once so humiliatingly bad at was all good.

With weekly lessons I learned valuable skills – life skills – such as how to hit through the ball and step aggressively into the court to try to win the point rather than assuming that I wouldn't. You have to believe in yourself and assert that belief, something I never could do as a child. We practised my inside-out backhand return of serve regularly, so that I could outsmart anybody who noticed that I am left-handed and hoped to beat me by serving down the T. If they thought they could avoid the strength of my cross-court forehand on the left-hand side, they had better think again. And as I relished every minor improvement, I felt a new sense of self-confidence growing in my body's strength, in my ability to win – not to mention the importance of wallowing around in the fun of pointless play.

Tennis is an intelligent game, where strategy and psychological advantage are as important as technique. You mustn't show any weakness, complain about the stiffness in your shoulder or the pain in your back because your opponent will sniff blood like a lion hunting a wounded impala. You have to talk yourself through each point and think about all the tiny ways you could change things when the game isn't going your way: more follow-through; move your feet quicker; drop the racket head further down your back or toss the ball higher when you're serving long or, worse, when you keep putting it into the net. With every one of these tiny points of focus the mind shifts down, concentrating, into the body, away from inhibition or insecurity, the very feelings that hold a girl back.

As a child, other than the boredom of standing around in the freezing cold, with an icy wind swirling about my bare knees as I occupied goal defence, the most inactive and isolated position on the hockey field, I don't remember playing much sport. But I could run fast and came home jubilant from a primary school sports day having run the hundred yards only a fraction of a second slower than the world record for women at that time. The teachers were excited and pleased for me. 'I think your running days are going to be limited,' my mother said sardonically, barely taking her eyes off the television screen, sitting in 'her' chair and squashing that achievement flat.

Sport wasn't cool for a teenage girl back then. Smoking was. Smoking a lot of dope was too, for my gang. So was losing your virginity, getting into pubs underage, wearing loon pants and clogs, shopping or shoplifting from Biba. What we didn't know was how important competitive sports are for building a genuine sense of one's own strength and self-worth. I only really found that in mid-life. The psychological lessons could have worked wonders in Bitchland, that place where girls go when they want to use the stealth missiles of exclusion and put-downs to feel better about themselves.

Men seem to sit more comfortably with the overt, playful competition of tennis, acknowledging each other's skills. Grown women expose something of the little girls they used to be. There are the cheats who shout 'out' when the ball is touching a line and then take umbrage, with sanctimonious indignation, when they are challenged. There are the lazy ones who never pick up the balls in that hiatus in group lessons when the basket has been emptied. There are the selfish ones – 'Who's volleying first, me?' – and the meanies – 'Ah, so you're just a fair-weather player then, are you?' I am the girl who bursts out laughing in the middle of a long point because she cannot believe the ball is still flying between rackets, or yelps with glee when she wins a point, irritating her opponents. For tennis has given me hundreds of hours of unadulterated happiness, for the first time in my life.

The essence of being a victim is that you become defined by everything that you cannot do. At primary school I was never allowed to feel like an equal member of a small gang, even though I was technically one of their friends. I tried to make them like me, taking presents into school, making up stories, lying even, in the hope that I would sparkle enough to impress them. At the age of eight I was using tactics that could never win; inadvertently, I was exposing even more of my weakness for them to prey on. They used to ask me to throw their apple cores away. I never said 'No, do it yourself' because I thought if I did what they said I could prove myself to be one of them. Make them like me. Accept me. I can still remember the smell of the browning, decaying core, ripped with teeth-marks and covered with saliva, as I carried it carefully by the stalk across the playground, weaving my way through groups of screaming children playing happier games to get to the rubbish bin. It became their daily thing, so that they could laugh and talk about me as they watched me walk there with everything they didn't want and then run back to them expecting praise and gratitude, which, of course, was never forthcoming.

The isolation and loneliness of that small girl who wandered between a home riven with the acrimony of divorce and terrible exclusion at school still haunts me sometimes. I never told my mother or a teacher, because the only thing that could have been wrong was with me. I had to work harder to make them accept me, not the other way round. I remember walking up the road to a friendly neighbour's house one day and asking if I could make a phone call. When she heard me ringing one of those girls to invite her over to my house for tea, the woman told me off for using the telephone for something so trivial. She wouldn't have known how making any phone call before 6 p.m. was forbidden in my house because it was more expensive, and that phoning after 6 p.m. felt like a very long time to wait for a little girl who believed that only phoning in that moment would help.

I have learned – the hard way – that the only person who can really help you is yourself. If you're losing in a game of tennis, blaming your opponent will not achieve a more positive outcome. Asking them to be kind and give you a few easy balls is going to be laughed off the court. You have to get cleverer, change tactics and surprise them. A large woman who is able to hit the ball really hard because she has strength in her arms? Hit the ball short with a cheeky drop shot, or to the left and then to the right and then angled to the left again so that she has to run for it. That's not cruel, just sensible. If you win the point a fresh confidence will sprout. You could win the next one too. If the sun is shining onto your opponent's side of the court, lob the ball high and often, so that she is blinded by the brightness. If she doesn't miss the ball she will certainly be unnerved by your change of tactic. Encourage her to make the same mistake again so that her self-confidence begins to turn. Whole matches can be won with psychology.

This game of competitive play can tell us much about how to win in life. It's important to expect to do well. Be aggressive, even. If you retreat defensively, your lack of confidence and your ineptitude will make you vulnerable. Over-sensitivity to the sharp barbs of your opponent needs to be seen off with banter – 'That would have been good if it wasn't out,' or 'Nice try!'

A good girl is supposed to be kind, enabling of others, nice – not expressing those natural human emotions of anger and selfishness. But in tennis there is a freedom within the white lines of the court to be me – sweaty and sunburnt, exuberantly lost in all the joy of play, competitive and crafty. I can shout obscenities with the frustration of doing something stupid or punch the air when I smash the ball back and kill its flight dead. But now, with such impaired physicality, I shuffle along like an old lady, hands on hips to protect my aching, fragile frame. I can feel myself being sucked back to that vulnerable little girl, that victim once again.

That is what I am struggling with. I am like that poor little me again. Feeling out of control, excluded and victimised. And it's not fair. I want to barge to the front of queues and say serve me first – 'I've got cancer.' I want to throw open the window at the top of the house and scream 'Why me?' I hear people laughing on the street or watch them running for buses and burn with jealousy at their freedom of movement, at how much they can take the physicality of being alive for granted. I start crying over the mildest problem – the GP's surgery losing a letter I need signed by a doctor, or being shunted around departments on the telephone. I snap angrily at passers-by who refuse to make room for me on the pavement. Emotions are close to the surface. I am angry, because life has suddenly truncated and changed radically, because I can no longer play tennis. I can feel the rest of the world spinning away from me, out of reach as a new sense of rejection, neediness and vulnerability takes over.

That same sense of heightened rejection I felt as a child I feel when people forget to call or keep a promise. When I am refused a massage because the therapist says she believes that, with so many chemicals in my bloodstream, moving them around 'could only make things worse', I feel like an untouchable. Isolated and alone.

I remind myself that this is me and my sensitivities. I have to egg myself on with the wisdom that I can't change the fact that I have cancer, but I can alter how I cope with it. Intellectually, I know that life isn't fair. I tell myself that other people around me are in all likelihood suffering from all sorts of torment, grief or pain too. I know that cancer isn't my fault. But that doesn't detract from the fact that this meteorite has hurtled out of nowhere and struck me down, inevitably turning all of my focus inwards.

The loss of the physicality is profound and sudden. My back is so stiff and sore from the fractured ribs that I cannot bend to pick things up, and seem to be clumsier than ever before, knocking things to the floor as I stumble about. Sometimes the muscles in my back go into agonising spasms, jerking my body in even more painful directions. Thankfully, my legs are solid and strong from decades of walking. I depend upon them entirely now, as I stand up slowly from a chair, or squat to retrieve the last remaining roll of loo paper that has dropped to the floor at the worst possible moment. I worry because as each day passes I feel my limbs growing weaker from underuse, and with such sudden weight loss my resilience is buckling, my stamina waning as I climb the stairs, one at a time like a child. It's as if the core of me is broken. I worked so hard, with regular tennis practice, building up strength and stamina in order to limit the frailties, the passivity and the depressive lows of growing older, only to find physical vulnerability here suddenly, smack, in an instant.

Independence vanishes too. I cannot put on my own socks, tie my shoelaces or lift a large saucepan. I cannot leap into the car and drive myself wherever I want to go. I feel myself sliding subtly over the line towards the point where I want others to do everything for me, volunteering for invalidity because it takes such an effort to do anything for myself. Again I am transported back to when I was a small child. 'Five bob if you can get through lunch without making a mess,' my father used to tease me. I never succeeded in earning that money. The rigidity of my back makes it hard now to get through a meal without spilling something on my clothes or onto the table. In the dead of night, when I lie awake and think about things like life expectancy, and how many people will come to my funeral and what they might say, those dark places that one is never allowed to visit in the light of day, I find myself clutching a small stuffed white rabbit with a pink ribbon around its neck, a present sent by a friend. It can be warmed up in a microwave to ease the aches and pains. But it's the comfort of this little soft presence in the palm of my hand that brings back memories of the dozens of soft toys that used to protect me in bed. Fred the owl and Ostrobogulus the clown and a white rabbit called Ambrosia kept me company through the solitude of night, just as this little rabbit does now while Christoph catches up on much-needed sleep beside me.

I used to pride myself on being so healthy, eating organic food and going to a weekly yoga class. I have never been on any kind of regular medication, surprising one GP who asked again and again, in sheer disbelief,

'You're really not on *anything*?' Now I rattle with all the drugs I have to take. A cocktail of eight Tramadol and eight paracetamol every day, just to bring the pain levels down enough to be able to move. A chemo nurse, usually Clare if I'm lucky, comes to my house every three weeks with a drip stand, a bag full of medical equipment and boxes of drugs. I am so very lucky, I tell myself, trying to go to the positive, that I don't have to sit in a hospital waiting room for hours and that I can lie on the sofa surrounded by comforts while I wait for her to come to me. She inserts a cannula into my arm for a thirty-minute drip of Avastin, a drug which helps to prevent the cancer forming its own blood supply, and one which is supposed to work well with the oral chemotherapy I take – ten pills of capecitabine each day. Two weeks on, one week off. I am so very privileged, I tell myself again. Avastin is generally not available on the NHS because it is so expensive, even though there are people with cancer who could benefit from it. Within days of taking the Avastin my blood pressure spiralled up and out of control and I was prescribed amlodipine to bring it down. One a night. And before Clare can leave she gives me one final jab in the stomach with a bone-strengthening drug call denosumab, which always stings the most. 'I don't want to hurt you,' she says every time. 'I know you don't, darling,' I say by way of comforting her.

After years of taking nothing stronger than coffee, the first cycle of drugs felt like being hit by a train.

Denosumab made my whole frame ache more than it had done before the treatment. Chemotherapy is like nothing anybody has ever taken before. It sends my body into spasms of nausea, the runs and shivering fear; it seems to dismantle every cell of my being to get at the cancer. Doing anything feels like walking through black treacle. Taste disappears, as does appetite. I have to force myself to take five mouthfuls of food just so that I can swallow the pills.

Suddenly I am an invalid, dependent on drugs to try to keep me alive. Suddenly all that history of trying to do the right thing by my body evaporates into a blaze of chemicals. I curl up on the sofa and want to die. And with free prescriptions as a cancer patient, I have enough morphine in the house to be able to do just that.

I sense how hard my family are finding it, the tears held back, the bags beneath the eyes as they watch me suffer. But I am the one who has to cope with the pain, the gruelling treatment and the fight to beat the bitch of cancer back. I am the one who has to stay home hugging a hot-water bottle, while Christoph is out playing tennis, or carrying on with all the things he loves to do. I know that they have to get on with their own lives and I am the first to say so and encourage them to go out. I am the one who has to bite my lip to stop myself from becoming the bitter victim. And I have to fathom gratitude for everything that they do for me rather than blaming them for all those minor faults that never used to matter before, for the responsibility for all of the chores I used to do is now theirs as I sit helpless on the sofa. And of course none of them are ever done exactly in the way I would like.

There is physical isolation too. I need a cordon sanitaire around my body to stop it from going into agonising spasms. No one touches me. I am a leper. I must be kept at a distance so that I avoid any germs people may be carrying, for chemo kills immunity as well as cancer. I cannot hug my husband at night, or sob into his shoulder as he tries to squeeze the sadness out of me because it hurts too much. I slide towards self-preoccupation, uninterested in what is going on in the world or the needs and views of others.

Such narcissism was a trait I always hated in my mother, who was always suffering from some mysterious ailment that needed sympathy. Nobody was ever as ill, as needy or as hard done by as she was. She could be quick to blame others – the Nazis, my father, her parents, even her children – for having compromised her life. I took her once to see her granddaughter perform the lead in a play when she was at RADA's Saturday school. I helped her carefully to the pavement and then she told me that she had read in a newspaper that morning about how much it costs to raise a child. 'A hundred and forty thousand pounds! That's what you owe me,' she said with a wicked glint in her eye.

And now here I am, in spite of having vowed never to be like her, equally vulnerable, trying oh so hard to squash the same ugliness in myself. I love life. My life. I want it back. Cancer has snatched away my health, my verve and my physical independence. I have aged ten years in ten minutes. I see my mother's gaunt and tense face whenever I look in the mirror. I feel just like her as I shuffle towards the kettle to make another cup of tea. She could drink gallons of the stuff, always with lemon. It is as if she has come back from the dead to inhabit my body, to remind me of how vulnerable she was in her own lonely suffering. I, like her, now feel blame and indignation rising when others haven't thought of me, as if this is somehow my right. And it takes Herculean efforts, battling through the chronic pain, nausea and sludgy exhaustion, to slap such loathsome self-pity back down into the deep black hole where it belongs.

I know that I have to find ways to do things for myself, however painful, however long the simplest task may take, even if it kills me. A victim expects the world to see only them, to adapt around their needs. A survivor adapts, creatively ducking and diving through an unequal, unfair world with their own independent route, their pride and privacy intact. Die, bitch cancer, I think as I force myself to swallow chemotherapy pills after breakfast and then again after supper, pushing them around the table like a child trying not to eat disgusting spinach and talking to myself as a mother would to that child – two gone, well done, just one more mouthful of food and then the third . . .

I realise that these levels of self-preoccupation could become obsessive. All that seems to matter to me now is me – timing the painkillers so that I can stay one step ahead of the spasms, whether or what to eat, endlessly washing my hands or using antibacterial wipes to reduce my vulnerability to infection. And then there are the side effects from the chemo to worry about. The list is long: anaemia, nausea, constipation, diarrhoea, loss of appetite, sore mouth and ulcers, tiredness, bruising and bleeding, hair loss, headaches, dizziness, chapped palms and soles of the feet, stomach pains, nosebleeds … There are pills that try to mitigate some of these symptoms, but mostly you just have to grin and bear it.

The literature and chemo nurses talk about 'flu-like symptoms', but when they are bad they feel more like bubonic plague or typhoid. And they don't mention the terrifying nightmares that make it hard to go back to sleep. I have been given a handy chart by the hospital, to help me to differentiate between the dangerous symptoms that require me to ring someone immediately and the less significant ones. Tingling in my fingers could mean I am about to have a stroke; chest pains and problems breathing could mean an imminent heart attack, for chemo can change the way the heart works. But then a tight chest could also be because of my fractured ribs, the shortness of breath because of mild anaemia. How am I to know the difference, I wonder as I stare at the chart, when I have never taken such toxic drugs before? How can I, a neurotic Jew who cannot help but believe that the worst will always happen because of our history, make a rational decision about the difference between the normal, to-be-expected side effects and the life-threatening ones that require an ambulance? When the charming and charismatic oncologist ran through the list of possible side effects on the consent form, 'death as a consequence of treatment' was one of them. Rare, he added with a faint smile.

'Feeling generally unwell' is in the 'mild' column of the chart, the 'moderate' column and also in the red column requiring an immediate call to the hospital. How can I not be feeling generally unwell, because of the shock diagnosis, the toxicity from taking so many pills, the pain in my limbs and muscles and the nausea? A tricky one to call, that. So I put the chart back into the drawer with the chemo and pretend I never looked at it. Side effects, shneide effects. I have no choice but to take the pills, so if a stroke takes me before the cancer, so be it.

Another critical symptom is a temperature of 38 degrees. That could mean infection and one that, with reduced immunity, might be harder to kill. We have never owned a thermometer. When the children were ill, I gave them Calpol if their foreheads were hot. If they didn't get better I took them to the doctor. There didn't seem much point in knowing exactly how high their temperature was. Cancer, however, has put a whole new shade of meaning on the need to know, so we bought a smart electronic thermometer that could be put into my ear. On day three of chemotherapy, when I felt shivery and 'generally unwell', I suggested we should probably be sensible and check my temperature. The only trouble was that we didn't know how to make the thing work. It flashed red with a measurement of 37.5 degrees in one ear and flashed green with 32 in the other. We struggled on with the technology, measuring everybody's temperature in an attempt to work out which reading was 'memory' being stored and which was genuine. When it reached 38 in the middle of the night and we rang, as requested, the kind person at the end of the phone said that she didn't think it sounded like I had flu, and anyway they couldn't consider any reading if I had also been clutching a hot-water bottle. We slumped back onto our pillows, relieved by the humiliation.

In mid-life we become survivors by definition. In all likelihood we will have lived through tragedy and trauma. Grief, illness, relationship difficulties, money worries, unemployment, family ructions, bringing up children or coping with childlessness are integral to the landscape of being human and alive, burdens we have to bear essentially alone. I have survived the collateral damage of my parents' divorce, the isolation of being bullied as a young child, the soul-searching of my twenties, the grief of losing friends young to drugs, working motherhood and caesarians. Even the first stage of labour with my first-born was achieved alone. When my waters broke we went straight to the hospital, where I was told I had hours and hours to go by a midwife and was put into a side room to sleep with two paracetamol for the pain. My husband was sent home. I got up regularly throughout the night to go to the lavatory and groan through contractions because I didn't want to wake the pregnant woman in the bed beside mine. It was only when I walked into the ward the following morning, feeling the baby trying to be born between my legs, that they examined me and found that I was fully dilated. Labour on two paracetamol.

So I know that I am the one who has to throw every ounce of energy and intelligence that I have into burying the bitch of cancer, for she is the bitchiest of bitches, just like I discovered at primary school, creeping up stealthily in the playground of life as she sucks vampirically at my strength to feed her own inadequacies.

The great wonder of mid-life is that I have exercised these muscles before. The experience of living through everything that has been before lays the foundations of resilience for what is to come: just as with every game of tennis, muscle memory builds. I know from everything that has gone before that I have the resources to stop myself from being yet another of cancer's victims, I tell myself as I whack a metaphorical tennis ball at the bitch's head and watch her face smash to smithereens, just as I should have done all those years ago with those presumptuous girls who dared to make me feel so small. And I know from everything that has gone before that between the great dark episodes there is always light, always an up after a down, love soothing loneliness and unhappiness, and that it is only by seizing those good moments when they happen that we can really flourish.

I know that I can fathom the same strength that allowed us to turn that last tennis game around, from losing to a decisive win. But I am going to have to dig deep, just as I did then, just as I did as a child, to come to terms with the poor prognosis and cope with the side effects of chemo. On some days my feet are so sore that I cannot walk, the tips of my fingers so tender that I cannot prise open the foil packets of painkillers and supplements, and even of the chemo itself. Sometime the nausea is so great that the smell of food makes me want to vomit. My dreams can be disturbing too, scary enough to keep me awake. But I will fight to beat this back, just as I have fought before. I will fight to live. And I will not be diddled out of that state pension, with the triple lock intact.

I will keep going, living as normal a life as possible so that others see me, not just my illness and my invalidity. Carrying on with the day-to-day, with the ordinary aspects of the life that I love so much, will be the ultimate triumph over cancer. You imagine before such a diagnosis that you would drop everything and do all those things that you have always dreamed of doing, ticking off the bucket list. But with a shortened life expectancy comes appreciation for the simplest things. Walking without fear. Running to catch a ball. There is so much to be grateful for – birdsong and the dawn chorus; the smell of a perfect rose; the rich blaze of fiery colour that comes with autumn in thin sunlight; the taste of lush strawberries and sweet mango; watching the sun set over the hills from the terrace of my brother's house in Italy; the enchantment of good novels, Bach and Mozart, films by Almodóvar and BBC costume dramas. I am so very lucky, I keep telling myself, just to be alive. I have the best medical care. I have the support of so many kind people. I may have to fight this disease alone, but I am held high in the arms of love from family and friends. I cannot imagine how anyone gets through this without that, or the money to take a taxi instead of grappling with the crush of public transport and the risk of picking up an infection.

While I mourn my sudden loss of physicality, I know that I will probably never be able to play singles in the way I used to again, fearlessly and aggressively, but I can look back and be grateful that I have dedicated a good decade of my life to such exuberant, joyful play. I do, however, nurture a very small ambition: that one day I might be fit enough to put on my own trainers, by myself, sling my tennis racket over my shoulder, put a can of balls and a bottle of water into my bag and walk to the park with Christoph. We will warm up from the service line, hitting the ball gently to one another, chatting about nothing much at all, before moving back to the baseline to hit some proper shots. We will then play together, in the way we have always played, with our own set of rules – if I win a single game I have won the set because of his superior male strength. I will laugh and squeal with joy as we spar like courting lovers, and he will look back at me with that twinkle in his eyes, for he has always taken such pleasure from seeing my joy in this game.

We will manage that. And we will resume gentle mixed doubles with dear friends. Even if we have to play as if we are old. I used to play regularly with a friend at Regent's Park and almost every week a group of four elderly men were there too. They hit the ball at each other with impeccable technique, never moving their feet as they punched the ball back and forth for the points alone. One of them even played in his normal shoes. Then they would break to sit down with a cup of tea and talk about their latest ailments before resuming play on whatever court was free. That is how I hope to be. We may need to dose up on painkillers and rub Voltarol into our aching muscles, and we may need the St John Ambulance on speed dial. But unless we move continually towards the light of what makes each day joyful, what on earth is the point, exactly, in being alive?

mediation

The psychological state of refusing to believe something because you don't want it to be true is a human coping mechanism. I recognise it after years of working as a family mediator helping couples to divorce or separate. It's terrifying for both of them, facing up to a future so profoundly different from the one they had imagined. Often, particularly when one of the pair is still in love and hoping desperately that the other will change their mind about leaving, it can take several sessions to get them both to begin to accept that their relationship is over. And that's if you have done a good job as a mediator. Often you haven't, and they leave the room in tears, vowing never to come back because some things are just too unbearable to hear.

It wasn't until after several meetings with my charming, charismatic oncologist that the truth slowly began to dawn on me: the treatment he was putting me through might never end.

'How many cycles do you have to have?' people would ask.

'Um ... he hasn't really said.'

When I braced myself to ask on my next visit to his office, he said: 'We have to keep beating it back, keep it in your bones. But sooner or later your cancer will find a way to work round the drugs and then we will have to try another treatment.'

He means line chemo. Even stronger stuff. My hair will fall out and I will grow pale and frail and look closer to the end, like some of the people in the Waiting Room of Death downstairs. I will have to wear one of those horrible turbans that says to the world I AM DYING FROM CANCER.

'Can the human body really take that kind of battering with constant doses of chemo?'

He nodded. 'Yes it can, sometimes for years, with breaks ... '

My refusal to really hear this horrible news, until the oncologist repeated it on several occasions, was reinforced by the fog of heavy painkillers and the shock of the diagnosis. But it wasn't just that. I didn't want to hear it.

A few years ago I had one of those light-bulb moments when a whole new path opens up and begs to be followed. I could do this, I thought as I interviewed for one of my books a family mediator about how she helps separating couples to minimise the impact on their children. I know what it is like to be a child of a prolonged and acrimonious divorce. I have the research in my head from years of writing books about family life.

Training to become a family mediator was a good idea. As a writer, I felt I had no real qualifications in anything. This work, I thought, could provide another income stream when the commissions and ideas dried up, security for the future, given that divorce and family breakdown is common. But something else, deep down inside, other than wanting to help people, was beckoning me.

The training wasn't easy. I had to strip away every assumption and accept that I knew nothing and needed to learn – always a good thing for a writer. I spent two years working on a hundred-page portfolio that was more arduous than any book I have ever written. I had to have exactly the right cases, which would demonstrate dozens of competencies, from active listening to pointing poor desperate people to potential services that might help them, even when I knew that, in all likelihood, they would not.

Mediation works on the principle that the best divorces are ones fashioned by the couple themselves. They know their children and what might be in the best interests of the whole family better than any judge or lawyer. The research shows that parents are more likely to stick to the agreements they make in mediation than those drawn up by separate solicitors, who often have (shall we say it like it is?) a tendency to be partial in their advice and to fan the flames of conflict in order to get the best deal for their client. That is, after all, their job.

Divorce may be a legal process, but court can be the worst place for the vast majority of families. Instead, with mediation, separating couples are encouraged to talk about the end of their relationship, so that both can come to terms with that new and unwelcome reality. Finances are fully disclosed so that a conversation about what might be a fair way to go forward, where individual needs are met rather than thinking of divorce and separation as a war that has to be won, can take place. Nobody triumphs in family breakdown. Everybody pays a price and it can be a very expensive one indeed, financially and emotionally.

Mediators try to coax unhappy and stubborn people down from their defensive positions so that they can see their situation more in the round. Mediators offer practical solutions and compromises as well as hope for a more positive future. And perhaps most importantly of all, mediators encourage people to take charge of the end of their relationship and determine their own conduct so that they can honour the love that they once had for each other and give priority now to the children, who are, for the most part, resilient and will in all likelihood be fine – provided the separation is handled well.

I found the work captivating. It felt like a huge privilege to be trusted by a couple at such a vulnerable and intimate point in their lives. Their stories were of the direst heartache – jaw-dropping accounts of infidelity, insensitivity, cruelty, betrayal, abuse – and unhappiness so profound that it seemed to pervade the whole room where they sat side by side, often unable to make eye contact, let alone speak to each other. I learned quickly how not to show shock when they revealed some dark, destructive aspect of themselves, or disapproval when one said something vile or abusive to the other: a fundamental principle of the job is that mediators never judge or take sides. If you do, you've lost them. Instead, you ask a question. And another. You always ask questions to try to open them up. How did that make you feel? Why did you feel the need to say or to do that?

Every session, an hour and a half, passed too quickly. Time vanished as I listened, trying to hear the underlying emotions of fear, 'the drop' when they let slip something important within their words. I tried and hoped to find some glimmer of light, a small compromise, an apology or an acknowledgement of their part in the breakdown, a twig of an olive branch of hope. The knots of relationship difficulties during separation are highly convoluted, like a mangled gold chain of a necklace. You can only tease out one tiny, thin link at a time, with difficulty. Once one section of the tangle is eased, others can follow, as the couple begin to trust the process, and you as their mediator.

I loved being part of a team, because my normal life of writing is a solitary pursuit. I loved being the least important person in the room, away from the egos of media folk, where people can lose touch with ordinary life. For it was always ordinary people sitting in front of me: bus drivers, police officers, accountants, teachers, stay-at-home mothers, airport security staff, social workers, a vicar – all struggling with one of the most seismic shocks of their lives. The end of a relationship that was supposed to last for ever is the end of dreams. It means the constant terrifying fear that you could lose your children, to the courts or to another land entirely. It often means losing your home, some of your most prized possessions and your quality of life, as finding two separate places to live is always more expensive than living together in one. And for one of the pair, it can mean a sense of profound rejection and loneliness, staring into a future without the person they still love.

On a good day, when I sensed there had been a breakthrough, when couples smiled as they left and carried on their conversation without me on the pavement outside, I punched the air with joy. On days when I could help new parents younger than my own kids, teenagers some of them, by encouraging their understanding of the fundamentals of good childcare and co-parenting, I felt genuinely useful. But on a bad day, when I was accused of wasting a client's time or felt myself being sucked in by one partner in an attempt to wound the other, when filling out a legal aid form to assess a single mother's disposable income on benefits pushed her just over the limit and therefore made her ineligible for free mediation, when I woke up in the middle of the night and realised what I should have asked to unlock something intransigent – on those days, I wanted to kick the walls and never do this work again. For these people haunted me. They followed me around Sainsbury's, on my walks, in my dreams: they were part of my daily life. They filled me with despair. I had failed them somehow; I could have, should have, done more to help.

Sometimes I felt it was asking too much of people. To be able to make rational decisions when they were at their most emotional, some even came close to temporary, delusional insanity because they were so distressed. I saw how money underpins everything, and that countless families struggle with not enough: itself a major trigger for blame, unhappiness, breakdown and divorce. So many people simply cannot afford to separate and yet that seems to them to be their only solution. I've listened to hundreds of arguments about who has or hasn't paid for what, and why money given by parents for deposits or home improvements needs to be reimbursed. I've wanted to shake fathers with good incomes for refusing to increase the maintenance they pay by fifty pounds a month just because there is no obligation to do so under the law. That's when it takes Herculean efforts of self-control not to accuse them of being petty bastards. Instead, you have to ask pertinent questions such as: would you feel the same way about denying your children something they might need if you were still together? The answer, of course, is usually no. Or silence.

When it comes to the children, the power politics can turn nuclear. Each parent is so desperate not to lose a single moment with their children, so determined to prove that they love and need them more, that they are prepared to spend a great deal of time and money arguing over the smallest things and refusing to back down. Why would you not want to let your child go to football or ballet on a Saturday just because it's 'your' day with them? Why wouldn't you let him bring them back at six instead of five on a Sunday night when he isn't going to be seeing them for the next ten days? Because they 'get tired/ need to have a bath and supper before school/ do their homework/ see me' just doesn't sound authentic when you know that this is all about control, winning this one small battle because the war is lost. Separated parents can become fixated by the minutiae of life, worrying about what their children eat, who they see and play with rather than remembering that the only thing that matters is that the young and entirely innocent feel able to move freely between the two people they love most in the world.

In the summer and autumn of 2015 I had two very tricky high-conflict cases. One was an arranged marriage with two children in a house that was falling down around all of them because neither would pay for essential repairs. They had barely talked to each other since becoming 'separated under the same roof' seven years earlier. The other case I picked up from court, where we sat, voluntarily and unpaid by the court, as mediators, on occasional days, hoping to be of help. An Australian mother of two small children was applying for the return of their passports so that she could take them home to attend a family wedding. The father had lodged the children's passports with his lawyers because he was scared they would leave the country and never come back.

I had five sessions with each of these two couples at roughly the same time, and it was gruelling. These four people seemed to be filled with such hate and desire for retribution that it was as if they were addicted to the conflict.

I began to feel as if all of the defences I had built around myself were being stripped away. I felt skinless. Oversensitive. As if I was being stabbed all over with tiny pin pricks, catapulted back to the impotency and vulnerability of my own childhood, as once again I absorbed a couple's rage, unhappiness and anxiety, and again felt burdened by an overwhelming sense that I was the one, and the only one, who had to sort it out.

Divorce had entered every cell of my being as a child and is still part of me, my story. I knew it was there. I knew it had tremendous power, determining the way I always put my family ahead of my needs as well as directing me towards the subject matter of my books. It seems incredible to me now, that foolishly, I hadn't realised that re-entering such a high-octane emotional zone was the deeper reason I was drawn to this work.

I took a break and discussed it with my supervisor who had kindly gone carefully through all of my paperwork, trying to assess what might have happened. She showed me the forms I had filled in when closing the cases. I had ticked the box saying that mediation had broken down. 'But I've read through all the session summaries and you did well, you really helped to move them on,' she told me. 'There were just some issues that you couldn't have helped them with because that's their job not yours.' In mediation terms the sessions had been successful, but I couldn't see that: I felt as if it was my responsibility to make them happier and I hadn't managed it.

When you are a child and your parents are at war with each other – continually, for years – the result is that you feel you have only one choice: to be good and not make life any more difficult. So I withdrew into the shadows. My parents told me different stories about why they had separated. He was (according to her) terrible with money, so bad that she never knew whether there was enough to feed us. He was a shit who had numerous affairs and wanted to leave. She was (according to him) neurotic, wanted to be single so that she could write and the divorce had been her idea. These conflicting versions were constant through much of my childhood, pulling me from side to side until I was old enough to be able to walk away from both of them.

As I grew up it seemed odd that they had ever been married at all. They were so different. My father was the eldest of five. They were a close-knit Church of England working-class family. His father was a window cleaner and they grew up in the slums of Victoria in London with little other than love. He was warm and generous, attracted perhaps by my mother's intellect, her glamorous foreignness and her love of the arts. My mother was more outspoken about their courtship. She told me she had fallen in love with his large, loving family, so very different from her own. They met at London University. He was the first in his family to go to university, on a scholarship; she gobbled up English literature and longed to be a writer. Perhaps this really was an attraction of opposites, with each looking for something they lacked in the other. It also has to be said that they were both very young and exceedingly good-looking.

I thought I had left that small girl who longed for peace between her warring parents behind. The girl who lived her life in the shadows. I used to hold back, watching and listening to their arguments on the phone through the cracks in the banisters when they thought I was asleep. I heard my mother threatening him with not being able to see us at all unless he paid her the alimony he owed. I remember time slowing down every Saturday afternoon as I stared down from the living-room window on the top floor at the street below, an agonising stillness as I waited and longed for my father's car to pull in. He was often hours late to collect us and sometimes he never turned up at all. I loved my father more than anybody else in the world. I took his side in the war, believing that he needed me to defend him because my mother's attacks on him could be so much more vicious than his on her.

We moved into a new flat and it was obvious my father was never going to live with us again. I wet the bed every night. Then I fell down the stairs and gashed my head on a nail and needed to have stiches. As my mother and I waited for a long time at the hospital she was affectionate and unusually calm, for my sake. It was from that night on that I stopped wetting the bed. This stands out as a rare tender moment, yet years later my mother quipped that I had stopped wetting the bed because 'You loved all the attention.' I was five years old.

I remember flashes of real happiness with my father, buried under his heavy dark grey overcoat with my brother in the back of an MG sports car as we blasted down the M4 towards Bristol with the roof down, squealing with delight every time we raised our heads into the wind. I remember the sparse casualness of his flats in Bristol and in London, regularly emptied by the bailiffs. I remember him teaching me how to make tea. 'How will I know when the water has boiled?' – this was before trip switches on electric kettles. He thought for a moment. 'It's when the sound gets very loud and then drops a little.' Always a musical man. My father had many weaknesses – making promises that he couldn't keep and a carelessness with money – but life with him felt liberating and fun, away from the gloomy strictures of my mother's routines. He cracked jokes, was warm, loving and kind. I could cuddle him; my mother felt bony and wasn't comfortable with physical touch. He told me once that his love for me was absolute and unconditional. My mother laughed at the absurdity of such a comment. 'Love is always conditional – what if you murdered somebody?' As if she thought I could. I was ten years old.

Days or weekends with my father usually meant going along with whatever he was doing, which usually meant accompanying him to timber yards. He loved carpentry, and could spend hours in his workshop hammering and sawing to make wardrobes, tables, toy boxes and shelving. Radio 3 or records would be played at top volume, through speakers he had erected in every room of the house, making it almost impossible to talk. Or he would play the piano, his fat fingers flying up and down the keyboard, repeating difficult chords and sections to try to get them right, his thick fringe bouncing up and down on his forehead from the exertions of practice. Sometimes he stuck his tongue out slightly and squeezed it between his lips with concentration. And he would hum too, swallowed up by the tune.

He could sleep for hours on a Sunday morning. My brother and I would jump onto his heavy, still torso shouting 'Tea and biscuits! Tea and Biscuits!' trying to wake him. When I was older and went to stay with him on my own, when he was living with his new girlfriend, I would make two cups of tea and creep into their bedroom, placing one cup beside each of their sleeping heads, trying not to wake them up but hoping desperately that they would. Sometimes I retrieved the cold cups of un-drunk tea and made fresh ones. And then waited for those to go cold too.

It was a lonely place, that first decade of life. Any child has very little power, but something fundamental is withheld to victims of a badly handled divorce – the ability to speak honestly. I knew that as soon as I revealed to one of my parents some new opinion, freedom, treat or restraint offered by the other, blame and rage, like petrol, would be chucked on the embers of their war. Or maybe it would be met with the silence of pursed lips, saying so much more. It was easier to hide under a veil of silence, to keep those two worlds separate and slide into the crevices between. And at really difficult moments, when, say, my mother shouted at my father down the phone that he was a selfish liar before slamming the receiver back onto its cradle with a ringing smack, I couldn't help but feel that it might be easier for everybody if I just wasn't there at all.

And that's part of the fabric of me now, for childhood burrows into our bones just like cancer. An unhappy childhood can never be exorcised. It oozes through every pore, influencing family relationships in millions of tiny unseen ways. If each of us has just one story to tell, then this is mine. In my job as mediator, was I also unknowingly negotiating with my own past, revisiting that landscape again and again in a pointless attempt to put it all right?

I cannot help but wonder now whether that emotional self-crucifixion unlocked the cancer. If we think of cancer as residing in every cell, the dark on the other side of light, then, to get it kick-started, something has to breathe life into it. Perhaps if I had left all that unhappiness buried in the dustbin of history where it belongs then this dark and parasitic pervading force would have remained tiny and dormant. The cancer began in my left breast, close to my heart. Perhaps if I had looked forward instead of back, found more joy and serenity in everything that I have, if I had found ways of seeing how my childhood had also given me strength and independence, rather than scratching that old itch until it was raw, then maybe, maybe, the cancer wouldn't have woken up at all.

I had sobbed with inconsolable loss into my pillow all those years ago because of a deep and constant unhappiness, because of a sense of powerlessness, an inability to change things in my family for the better as well as a constant longing for the father I adored. In the first few weeks of being diagnosed with cancer, I sobbed daily with sheer despair, wailed even, with the same sense of inconsolable loss. My life, the life I had imagined for myself, was suddenly over. I couldn't control the cancer or make it go away. Did this new extreme pain mean that it was spreading? And where would it go next – my liver? My lungs? The closest organs to the breast or somewhere a little further away like my brain, destroying my ability to think or write clearly? I cried without stopping for three whole days when the penny dropped that I was never going to be better; I lay wounded on the sofa and grieved the future – grandchildren, travel to exciting places, happier times in a prolonged old age.

The tears of childhood and being diagnosed with an incurable cancer are tears of heartache, deeper than the pain of unrequited love, even. They are born of isolation, of a sense that one is utterly alone in this world. I cried when I said goodbye to my father as a child, harbouring a deep fear that I might never see him again. And I cry now with every goodbye, for every moment feels more pertinent. Will this be the last time that we meet, or that I am able to say happy birthday to this person I love? Will this be the last New Year's Day, now that it is also the first with such qualified hopes for the future? The tears come suddenly and without warning, when I feel overlooked or overwhelmed, when I feel that this wretched illness stands between me and those I love, when I can see the sadness in others' eyes forcing a vacuum of disconnection between us, when Christoph can no longer kiss me or see me as the sexual woman he once desired simply because everything, literally everything, is now qualified by this cancer that stalks me with the spectre of loss.

It's s battle, and battle is the right word, however un-PC that might be. And as a child I had to fight too, just to carve out a small space away from the divorce, a place of peace where resilience could flourish with reading, fantasy and sweets as I struggled with something I couldn't have understood then – the ordinary human inadequacies of my mother and father.

If cancer hasn't flourished because of the way that mediation took me back to the grief of my childhood, then where did it come from? I cannot help but ask the question. Perhaps it's the environmental toxins that hover in the air, infiltrating the waters of North London with poisons that my liver can no longer cope with. Perhaps I should have been more determined to eat only organic food and clean the house only with organic products. Why didn't I install an industrial water filter in our house? Why did I eat so much sugar when I knew I was overweight, when I knew that the resulting inflammation can cause a plethora of diseases? Why did I strive to achieve as a working mother instead of relaxing into the daily flow of looking after children, who move at a slower and healthier pace? Or maybe it was something much simpler that caused this misery – mercury in my mouth. I remember endless trips to the dentist as my teeth grew crooked and overcrowded my mouth. I had numerous extractions, painful braces and fillings. Was that it?

But you can't live a good life constantly looking back over your shoulder. A fundamental principle of mediation work is that what's past is past, what's done is done and cannot be undone. It can only be learnt from. I know intellectually that cancer isn't my fault, just as my parents' divorce wasn't my fault either, but the self-blame continues. Why didn't I go to the doctor when I first started feeling that itchiness in my left breast? Why didn't I read the small print on that last mammogram letter, saying that some breast cancers cannot be detected by this type of scan? But who does, after you have sighed with relief at the opening sentence, which is that the breasts are clear?

I walked away from my parents' relentless battles when I left home as an independent seventeen-year-old and never went back. I decided I didn't care any more and didn't want to know. I tell myself that I have to do the same now. It's utterly pointless indulging in any form of blame. My parents found it hard to do the right thing by their children but they didn't know any better; nobody did in the sixties. Few people got divorced then and there was no research or advice as to how to limit the damage to the young.

There is no need to shoulder blame for getting cancer either. All I can do is to try to face it head-on. Divorce and cancer are grenades thrown into the heart of family life, affecting everyone. Few families get through life without some sort of tremor sending them spinning, faster and faster, towards implosion unless you can find ways to talk about it. So I am determined to replace the silence I clung to as a child with frankness. We talk about this grenade, often. I tell my family that I have no intention of dying soon and that they have to get on with their own lives rather than worry about me. I tell them that they only need get concerned when I stop being bossy or difficult. We have to keep talking about it, and even laugh sometimes with the blackness of it all.

I found mediation attractive because it is a powerful way to help families help themselves, by placing the responsibility on the grown-ups. 'You have an opportunity now to make this as pain-free as possible for your children if you handle it well,' I used to say to parents whenever they expressed worries about their kids because of the separation. With tiny incremental steps, confidence in their own ability to face an uncertain future grew. Over the weeks I saw tears turn to smiles as parental relations improved and they began to approach their domestic problems differently. I have to do the same for myself now. I have to take responsibility and find my own way through this jungle of shock and change. 'I will beat this,' I tell my family over and over again to pull us all back together, forcing myself to be kinder, more attentive and loving even though I feel like death. I tell them that I have to find ways to change my life, to change whatever may have caused this parasite to grow inside my body, in order to live. Whatever it takes, I will do it.

And key to that has to be finally drawing a line under the past, just as I have told dozens of miserable couples over the years. Training as a mediator has helped me to understand something of what my parents lived through when we were children. As a child I could only see it from a child's point of view. I now see that going back into the dark den that has defined so much of my life to slay the dragon that lives there one last time might well have been useful as well as painful. My parents, locked into conflict as their prime defence mechanism, refused to climb down because they were miserable, vengeful and terrified of what might lie ahead. In mediation I saw how the despair and sense of loss was far worse for many separating parents than it was for their children.

I can see too how like both my parents I am. They valued learning, music, literature and the arts as much as good food, and it is these that nourish me most now. Both were fighters, as am I. My father came from a poor working-class family and educated himself with books, Bach and ballet. My mother managed well as a single mother, equipping us with everything we needed as growing children, from food to music lessons – and on next to no income. She carved out a successful career as a novelist and published a 'seminal' book on feminism in 1970 called *Patriarchal Attitudes*. She helped to define the 'second wave' of feminism, and because I was thirteen when it came out, and my mother was all over the media talking about sexual equality, I grew up believing in the value of feminism; I never had to find it as an explanation for a woman's lot, as so many others did.

I am proud to carry them both with me, under my skin. My father's dry sense of humour, his love of Christmas, his warmth and generosity. My mother's refusal to be sidelined, her strong moral compass and her tenacity. She told me that she refused to speak at school, having arrived in this country as an 'enemy alien' aged seven, until she could utter a perfect English sentence and so would not stand out as strange.

Perhaps it is that same dogged determination which keeps me going through this hell. For most of her life my mother struggled with compromised health – chronic eczema and an addiction to cortisone, regular digestive problems and infections, acute anxiety and a dampened mood. I understand now how her physical problems must have hammered away at her optimism. But she kept going through it all. She went to the doctor regularly and demanded tests when she was sent home with an inconclusive diagnosis. Perhaps if I'd been a bit more like her, instead of doing everything I could to differentiate myself from her by rarely going to the doctor at all, I would have demanded tests too. I was perhaps too much like my father, who rarely went to see a doctor either. He insisted he just had irritable bowel syndrome when the stomach cancer that would kill him was eating him up inside. I miss them both: but it is comforting now that I am so ill to feel them close by. It isn't the unhappiness I experienced with them that rises to the surface now, it's their qualities and the love they had for me.

I don't deny that it has been important to revisit those hurts one last time, but now I have to bury them for good to age well, embracing every last joyful moment, unhindered by that past. When mediation becomes so locked that it is doomed to fail there is one lifeline. The mediator throws the problem straight back into their faces: 'So what are *you* going to do if you can't reach an agreement here? Because it really doesn't matter to me what you do. I walk out of here and get on with the rest of my day.'

And that's what I plan to do now. That has to be the key to living mid-life well, whether or not you are ill: turn back to take one final look at all those regrets and then face forward. I have also learned from my work as a mediator how important it is to be able to walk away from something into which I have invested huge amounts of time, money and energy. That's not a loss, but a gain. It opens up the space for a very different future. It has been a privilege to be allowed to revisit the landscape of my own childhood from a different per-spective – colonic irrigation of the soul. But cancer has also shown me that you don't have to keep bashing away at something just because you began upon a journey that you thought would lead you into a different direction. I didn't have to mourn my upbringing any longer, just as I didn't have to do this draining work with miserable separating couples. I didn't need to put myself through this pain any longer. I could give it up, and not feel a weak failure for doing so. So I stopped mediating, just like that.

With the same sudden decisiveness, in less than an hour, I chucked out all the research I have used for my books that has been gathering dust in the office for twenty years. We needed the shelves now for other things, for what matters today. I turn to my wardrobe. I have shrunk from a size fourteen to a ten; my clothes hang so large on my frame that I look even iller. So, in a matter of minutes they were packed up and round the corner at the charity shop. It was all so easy. All these things that had been useful once were now drains. I didn't have to keep them.

I remember my father once telling me that I had to be careful, that I felt others' pain too deeply and needed to toughen up and make sure that I found my own joy in life because deep sadness can cause cancer. He actually said cancer. Ironic now I have it, but a coincidence probably. He couldn't have known. But what he was really telling me was that it was important to move on, to get over the unhappiness of my childhood so that I could find more pleasure in my own life. Just as separating couples have to find a way to accept that their future might be poorer or lonelier than they had expected, I have to toughen up and find a way to accept that cancer has struck for whatever reason and that it has brought compromises that have to be lived with. I have to accept that these strong and toxic drugs could be prolonging my life and so have to be taken, possibly for ever. Now, a little late in the day perhaps, I think I might be finally learning how to achieve what my father had wanted for me all those years ago: how to ride above all the shit that an ordinary life throws up. What an irony that it is bitch cancer, which will probably end my life, that I have to thank for that.

the beach hut

A wooden hut measuring ten foot by eight and painted
a vivid turquoise with bright pink stripes offers a very
private place of peace. Not so much a room of one's own;
more a bolt-hole, somewhere to escape to when things
get too much, for mindlessness instead of mindfulness,
a place to disconnect from the hard shoulder of life. For
years, 'I am going to the beach hut' became shorthand for
'I need to run away but you will know where I am so no
need to worry'. I stripped possessions back to the basics.
The books I needed for work. Clothes for the predicted
weather. A small bag of nutritious food. A large bottle of
water. And then I would set off from the city, exuberant
and liberated by the knowledge that with solitude and
isolation my anxious, over-active mind could rest for a
while.

On clear days I sit outside the hut and watch tankers

on the horizon heading slowly for Portsmouth past the eastern tip of the Isle of Wight, and the small white sails of yachts zig-zagging across the Solent. The sun hits the beach at mid-morning and then crosses steadily over the sea, charting the preciousness of time before it sets over the mainland beyond the cliffs of Dorset. I can sit here for hours watching the tide recede, the white surf growing smaller as the sound of the waves evaporates into the wind, the blue sky above streaked with wispy cloud. Land, sea, sky and time merge and melt into each other. This is an exquisite, moving watercolour, shimmering with every shade of yellow, blue, grey and white. As the vast, dark sea is sucked back into itself, sand banks and rock pools emerge, encouraging small children to venture out over the new shore with buckets and spades to look for shells and crabs. And then the tide turns, slowly swallowing up the beach again.

In winter, and for much of the autumn, the beach is often cold and windy, deserted save for the odd intrepid dog-walker. Then the hut is a perfect shelter. I sit at a table pretending to work and stare through a small square glass window streaked with sand and mist at windsurfers riding the waves in wetsuits. I boil the kettle on a butane gas cooker for a warming mug of tea and line up my rations for the day on the tiny doll's-house counter – an apple, a cheese and tomato sandwich, nuts and a precious bar of chocolate – a treat to look forward to and savour slowly. When will that be? And when the sea sounds soothe like a lullaby, a sun lounger is the perfect bed to doze on, wrapped in a blanket as the wind whistles around the asphalt roof and rattles the shutters.

In spring and summer the beach buzzes with the sounds of happy children, running in and out of the huts playing hide-and-seek. Windbreaks and umbrellas punctuate the yellow sand with stripy colour. I sit outside, proprietorially, as young couples, teenagers bunking off school, families with small children and coach parties of day-trippers struggle past, kicking off their shoes, trying to push buggies laden with cool bags, rugs, picnic hampers, disposable barbecues and ball games through the deep sand. Some, curious, wander in front of me so that they can peek into the hut. Then, just a few hours later, the beach begins to empty again. That's when it belongs just to me and the seagulls that walk casually about the sand, pecking at what has been left behind.

We all need a bolt-hole, time to be alone. When my children were young I used to go to the beach hut to escape the constancy of the demands of working motherhood. I had to keep it all together, and be seen to be keeping it all together. No shouting at the children. No drinking before their bedtime. No moaning about our lot. 'Just tired,' we working mothers say when we are asked what's wrong. 'You're always tired,' my youngest used to reply, wanting me to be livelier, happier.

It felt to me then that the only way was to struggle on, fitting everything in somehow. Children have to be got to school, calls have to be answered, money has to be earned, washing has to be loaded into the machine or taken to the launderette, food has to be bought and cooked, packed lunches have to be made, distraught, angry teenagers have to be talked down, brought back into line or comforted. And then we wonder why our temper suddenly zooms from apparent calm to acute, murderous rage in just a few seconds. Who is this crazed and demented woman? Often I did not recognise myself.

Knowing I could escape felt so exhilarating and essential. I knew I was lucky. Driving just a little bit too fast with the windows down and singing along to the Rolling Stones or Abba at top volume made me feel younger and freer. The beauty of the flowers in the hedgerows, the trees in the green fields beyond: all seemed to make my heart sing again with gratitude that I had somewhere to run to. And when I got to the coast, parking on the grass behind the hut, and ran out onto the vast expanse of the beach, the simple excitement of not knowing whether the tide would be in or out, whether the wind was up and the waves high or the sea calm and placid filled me with childlike wonder. Then there was the welcome sanctuary of the hut itself. For twenty-four hours I would only have myself to care for, to replenish, so that I could go back and be a nicer person. It would take just four hours of watching the sea, or fussing around making a cup of tea and sweeping out the sand carefully from the corners before I began to feel whole again, and miss home.

In this beautiful place every day and every aspect of the view is subtly different, shaped by the changing weather, the time of year, the colour and ferocity of the sea, the strength of tumultuous storms and the searing wind as it hurls sand against the dunes, sculpting the land. And yet because the scene is always somehow the same too, it offers me a sense of constancy through change. I watch this mesmerising moving picture soften when the light fades with such gentleness I begin to soften too, more at ease with the change and uncertainty that seems to rock my world.

The hut was bought with money inherited from my grandmother, money I had no idea what to do with until the chance of buying this hut came my way.

My mother's family left Berlin suddenly in 1939, abandoning their home, their possessions and my mother's grandparents on both sides of her family. None survived. My mother was seven years old and that upheaval was traumatic for her. I think I only really understood how much she longed for her severed childhood when I took her back to Berlin with my own children. We were staying in Charlottenburg, where they had lived before the war, and she seemed content, relaxed and at one with her surroundings as she stared up at the tall linden trees on the street where she used to live. Though she was in her seventies it was as it she had regressed to being seven again, seeming almost to skip along the pavement, picking hot roasted almonds out of the paper cone we'd bought for her with an expression of happiness on her face I had never seen before, or saw again.

The summary of their story is this: her father, my grandfather, was arrested in Munich, where he was on a visit for work, on Kristallnacht and taken to Dachau. My grandmother found a channel through which she could bribe the guards for his release; it involved buying shares in a Chilean shoe factory, which my grandmother assumed did not exist until the share certificate turned up after the war. She then waited anxiously for three weeks for him to come home and when he returned he was stick thin, with scarlet fever. My mother remembered his shaved head. My uncle told me that he believed Grandpa had been released because they didn't want the disease to spread through the camp, and that the bribe had been used for my family's exit visas from Germany. My mother believed otherwise, that if he had come down with scarlet fever at Dachau he would have died there.

While my grandfather was in the camp at Dachau my grandmother booked passage on a boat from Hamburg to Thailand, the only country that would accept Jews in 1939 without entry visas. Luckily perhaps, they missed the boat because my grandfather was so ill. Visas for Britain arrived soon afterwards and they flew out of Tempelhof airport, leaving both sets of my mother's grandparents behind: they refused to leave.

The efforts of my grandmother, first in securing her husband's release from Dachau and then in getting all four of them to safety in England, saved their lives. My grandfather joined the British Army, and as a native German speaker was put to work as a translator for those interrogating prisoners of war. He was advised, as a Jew, to change his name in case of capture but he refused and marched as Emil Unger all the way back to Berlin with the Allies in 1945. It was the only time he ever returned to his homeland.

This is the history, the extraordinary grit of the two people, the grandparents I loved as Nana and Grandpa. As a child, I knew little of their dangerous and terrifying history other than that they had left Berlin in 1939 because of the war. I did not then understand the courage they had to muster, nor the heartbreak, homesickness and trauma, because it was never talked about. They simply did their best to be loving grandparents, making jokes, handing out sweets to keep us going on long walks or extra pocket money to spend on holidays, and bought us bottles of delicious bitter lemon – to be savoured slowly, because we were only ever allowed one with lunch.

It is only now that I wish I could have had just one real conversation with my grandfather about his experiences during the war. But he died of a heart attack when I was fifteen. My grandmother lived on for many more years and we were close. Even so, talking about those times was avoided. 'It is best to forgive but never to forget,' my grandmother replied when I once tentatively raised the subject of Nazi Germany. But how can one ever really forgive that?

They had been 'lucky' and yet the horror hung in the air, in everything that wasn't being talked about because it was 'best to move on'. Their home and possessions were modern, born of the G Plan design revolution; nothing of German origin was ever brought into the house. But other things spoke of their lost homeland, like my grandmother's deliciously buttery cabbage and her cauliflower cheese, which seemed to taste cheesier and with more cauliflower flavour than any I have ever eaten since. On Christmas Eve my grandfather lit the tiny red candles on the Christmas tree and we sang 'Silent Night'. They rarely spoke German, but they couldn't help but sing this beautiful carol in their mother tongue.

I grew up knowing, instinctively, that it would be too painful for them to speak about those times so it was better not to ask. Now, as an adult with grown children and, having read enough accounts by other Jewish refugees, I can begin to understand how deep and far-reaching was the mourning for the life and the family that had been lost. My grandparents and my mother had not been allowed to say goodbye. No funerals. No memorials. No counselling to help them cope. Instead, the six million who died have been carried inside those who 'survived'.

Holocaust damage ran through my family, distorting the natural balance of relationships, and my mother suffered particularly badly. She said that her mother turned cold and vengeful when they got to Britain, taking out all her rage for what had happened to them on her daughter. I think, knowing them both, that Nana was simply exhausted from her efforts – getting them out of Nazi Germany alive and then living through five long years of the war. Nana had herself baptised here – as a precaution, no doubt, but my mother maintained that this was a disguised anti-Semitic act. She had thought of herself as German first, not Jewish, and they had been deeply assimilated into Berlin life. If Germans could do that to Jews, then perhaps there really was something wrong with them.

The loss of her home, her native language and the love of her own mother tormented Eva for much of her life. As she grew older, most things for her seemed to relate in some way back to her childhood. She could never really put it behind her. Perhaps nobody who has lived through such an experience can. The Holocaust is, and continues to be, such a powerful force that a vast black hole seems to suck all of us back to that time whether we were there or not. Persecution of such magnitude tumbles through the DNA of family life. It distorts and corrupts the normal and essential building blocks of love, managing risks and adversity. I cannot help but feel a responsibility to carry that history with me too, so that we never forget, just as my grandmother told me. It's a delicate balancing act – how to honour what they lived through without allowing it to burden the present with paranoia and insecurity. The feeling of the need for retribution remains strong.

I am aware that the calm the beach hut brings me is linked to that turbulent past, and not just because it was bought with money left by my grandmother but because I have been here with them. The hut sits at the end of an estuary that we used to sail with my grandfather. He never looked happier than when he was in that boat with the wind in his face, hand on the tiller. They had owned a boat in Berlin, which they used to sail on one of the lakes. After the war, my grandfather rebuilt their lives with a new and successful business. They designed their ideal retirement home – a purpose-built bungalow in Sussex with a glorious view over the South Downs – and bought a boat, which was moored a mile or so away from the hut, at Bosham.

On weekend visits and in the summer holidays Grandpa would take us sailing. My brother and I stood on the back seat of his Ford Cortina, sticking our heads out through the open sunroof as the car wound slowly through the country lanes towards the coast. A small ferry dropped us at the yacht, which was built of the creamiest wood with two tiny beds in the hold. We clambered on board, pulled up the anchor and tacked down the estuary towards Hayling Island until the Isle of Wight came into view, then we would turn back, past the sand dunes and inlets I now walk along. Sometimes we would throw down the anchor and, looking out to sea, munch on the sandwiches that my grandmother had made. When we set off again I would lie on my stomach on the hull watching it cut through the waves below while catching at the water with my fingers as the wind forced the boat to keel sideways. Possibly it's that memory that makes me love watching the waves crash onto the shore now. I hear the noise of sail ropes clanking against masts as I walk up the same estuary and the sound takes me instantly back to that childhood with a tingling, visceral hit.

I salute my grandparents every time I drive past the turning to their village off the A3, a gesture of respect for what they lived through and gratitude for what they have given me. Life. The beach hut. A history of courage, survival, difference, and the wary, wily, knowledge that comes from knowing that once persecution has entered your gene pool it never leaves. It burrows deep down and shoots out warning signs. It could happen again. Money needs to be saved for a running-away fund, a suitcase packed in the hall. I know that anxiety can become my middle name unless it is battered down by sensible reason. Uncertainty is the name of the human game even as we try to root our worlds with status, possessions and purpose. After what my family lived through, a little cancer isn't going to beat me.

Now that my grandparents and my parents are dead and their homes, my childhood homes, have been dismantled, the hut feels like a last bastion of retreat, but it sits on shifting sands. It could be washed away. It is on the brink of instability, just as we all are whether we are healthy or ill. Being there for a few hours reminds me that there really is only today. Though I have a past to remember and a future to define, all is humbled by the dynamic force of nature. But here I can choose to sit back and enjoy the view rather than scan the horizon for new threats.

Back in London, with cancer, I think about the beach hut often. I long for it as I lie back over the hot-water bottle on the sofa. I know how healing it is, how it could offer a very special sanctuary, solitude, a place for reflection, a link back to my grandparents' powerful and humbling example of triumph over adversity, if only I could get there on my own. Driving is impossible and I am not strong enough even to be able to lift the wooden bar that locks the hut. My fingers are sore too from the chemo, the skin so thin. I can't race to my bolt-hole at the very moment when I need it most, for that clear space to think myself into a very different future and feel more at ease with it. The weather this autumn has been glorious too – days and days of warm low sunshine; there would have been spectacular sunsets over the sea. I stifle jealousy with reason and the thought that at least others can enjoy it when I see pictures on Facebook of Sal, my beach hut 'sister' (the friend I bought the hut with), relishing the beauty and peace of our very special place.

After losing everything but each other and their children, my grandparents cherished their luck and established new roots in a Sussex field, which my grandmother tamed into a beautiful garden. Past tragedies and loss meant they enjoyed even more the pleasures such as sailing, holidays and the arts. My grandparents knew how to age well. What role models. I take strength from them and set my mind to progress and to getting back to something of how I used to be – even if that means sitting at the hut with others until I am strong enough to go alone.

Mid-life is a curious place: a bit like standing on the top of a tall hill that it has taken decades to climb. You can look back at where you have been, at the deep and distant past and everything that has happened, all the missed, wrong turnings, all the beautiful landmark moments, because there is so much past now to assimilate. And then you turn at the top of the hill and look down to the other side, to where you're heading. Death lies somewhere down there, coming closer with every year. The question now is which path will lead you there. What now seems to matter is making sure that you stick to the long wiggly one with all sorts of interesting detours along the way. Mid-life is precious because it feels so uncertain, full of possibilities once again – in my case and others, freed from the responsibilities of caring for children and ageing parents.

What we want to avoid are the more direct routes to death, or the cul-de-sac of illness. I find myself in that dreaded cul-de-sac and now, surveying things from the top of that hill, the past suddenly feels wasted and the future down the other side seems very short indeed. But the view, oh the view of life all around is so spectacular. It has never looked so beautiful, so transient, so precious. I want to capture every tiny detail in the camera of my mind. It's easy to see now the folly of past mistakes and my tendency to play it safe. Risk has always been difficult, perhaps because of what my mother and grandparents lived through. Perhaps I have been pre-programmed to select the safest route through life, which is why the beach hut feels like such a delicious aberration. It felt so reckless and extravagant at the time; now I can't imagine life without it.

We bought it on a whim, with old friends who live near the coast. Sealed bids had to be entered by the following day. We had no idea what to offer and probably paid way too much. But something deep inside told me that we had to have it, in spite of all the uncertainties ahead. We knew that weather and climate change could sweep it away. Indeed, for two successive winters it has been flooded and we have been unable to open the door because we couldn't even get to it. Would our friendship survive shared ownership? And why buy a hut that you aren't allowed to sleep in? All perfectly good reasons to say no, except for the fact that the whole point of the hut is its exposure to the uncertainty of the elements, the sheer frippery of it, money spent on an indulgence, on something unnecessary just for the pleasure of it and it alone. Because that hut is the only folly of my life, it has become even more precious.

We are all so much more on the edge of things than we want to believe and there is nothing like a beach, where the land meets the vastness of the sea, to remind us of that fact. Where fun can meet tragedy as a child gets washed away by the current on a rubber ring; where thousands of refugees get swallowed whole every year as they try to reach safety just as my mother and her family once did. All of us are equal on a beach in our vulnerability.

A beach is democratic. It reduces everyone to the same small speck of humanity within a massive landscape. A beach is a playground where age doesn't matter; it is offered up freely by nature to enjoy. We plunge into a parallel world where past memories of childhood and being with our own children merge and surface in the present. We know instinctively how to be on a beach, how to lose our senses in the feel of sand between our toes, the wind in our hair. How to write names or messages of love in huge letters with spades or draw pictures of mermaids and pretend that seaweed can be long curly locks and shells are nipples. We know how to dig holes and bury our legs, or create elaborate castles with flags and moats, which fill with the incoming tide before collapsing beneath the weight of the waves.

We know how to play bat and ball over an imaginary net or beach cricket with no real boundaries. We know how to jump the waves and squeal as the cold of the sea creeps up around our stomachs before plunging in . . . to what? The great exhilarating and dangerous dark of a vast, uncontrollable sea beneath our tiny, paddling feet.

And yet, there is a wider order, a regularity, a rhythm and circle of life which is way, way bigger than any of us – the regular magnetic force of the earth, the pull of the moon that controls the tides. All out of our control. That is the only certainty.

Our hut has provided a refuge for grief and heartbreak; a place to revise for exams or work, a love shack for budding romances as well as a place for laughter and parties, for people to gather together and share food, buckets and spades and stories. For in the end that is what sustains us: the connections we forge with one another, and the wider extended family beyond ties of blood. The beach hut roots us through time simply by being there, whether or not it sits on shifting sands. It is a fulcrum through time and generations. It's a place where my girls can go in the future to be with me long after I am gone. For what else matters in mid-life, when ambition and opportunity begins to fade, other than handing on some valuable torch, some tiny and meaningful legacy to those we love which will connect them back to those we have loved. That's a chain that cannot be broken.

One day I hope to sit there with my grandchildren and tell them stories of my own, how we used to sail down the estuary, how my grandparents had to escape from a country far away for safety and found it here. I will feel their tiny hands in mine as we paddle in lagoons that open up when the tide is out to look for shells. We will sit together and enjoy ice cream and then watch the sun go down over the sea. But until that time I will be content if I can just manage to get there on my own, for that blissful solitude which has kept me sane all these years. I know that the day will come, possibly too soon, when I will be so frail, and hopefully so old, that I won't be able to get there at all. Then I can see myself lying back on the pillows, eyes closed as I imagine myself there, for the pictures from that hut are so vivid they live on in my mind. That is such a gift. So yes, that will be enough. I am so very proud of taking that leap into the dark to buy that little shed on a beach.

tales from the hyperbaric
oxygen chamber

'Give up sugar and contact Patricia Peat. She will really
help.'

Jerome Burne, a friend and a health journalist,
answered my email with 'HELP!' typed into the subject
box with this message and he was right. She has helped
to change my life for the better.

Patricia Peat worked as a chemo nurse for fifteen years.
She noticed that people who used so-called alternative
methods while they were on chemotherapy or radiother-
apy seemed to cope better with the treatment and live
longer, so she set up her own consultancy helping people
to do just that. Smart woman.

I can book a telephone conversation with her whenever
I need an extra voice to answer questions, another form of
expert support. At first, I was so dazed and confused by

the diagnosis and the wealth of drugs flooding through my body that I found her battering of positive advice overwhelming. During our first call I could also have sworn I could hear her eating her lunch at the other end of the phone, while I sat dissolved on the floor, nothing more than a puddle, my life scattered all around me. After an hour's consultation she emailed me a sixty-page attachment on what I could do to help myself, complete with academic research papers on triple negative breast cancer. It was so terrifying to read I could only manage a page or two at a time before I slammed the computer shut in horror. But as the shock began to fade I consulted this document more and more and found it really helped.

In that first phone call Patricia asked me if I lived close to Walthamstow. I did. 'Great, that is the best news. Are you mobile? Not yet? OK, well as soon as you are, get yourself up there for some oxygen therapy. That will help your bones to heal.' So I hobbled up to the GP surgery to get my form from MS Action signed, confirming that I was a cancer patient and could therefore join this remarkable little charity. They have been providing oxygen therapy for MS sufferers for nearly forty years, but accept cancer patients for oxygen therapy at a higher fee. And then as soon as I was able, in February 2017, Christoph drove me up to an industrial estate just off the North Circular, where, nestled between Screwfix and Photomart, sits MS Action. This was where things started to improve.

MS Action is staffed by volunteers. They raise money through raffles and selling donations displayed on tables at the entrance. People with MS can go there for physiotherapy to help ease their symptoms or simply to have their toenails cut. There is also the hyperbaric oxygen chamber, a large metal cylindrical dome with tiny porthole windows and lots of fishes painted on sea-blue walls. Inside are six armchairs, where people with MS and other conditions sit for ninety minutes wearing a mask, which brings in pure oxygen on one side and eliminates the waste breath on the other, during which time the pressure inside the dome is reduced. 'Taking you down to twenty-four feet,' as the 'driver' tells us over the intercom at the beginning of each session. With reduced pressure, blood vessels expand and oxygen is more easily absorbed into the cells of the body.

As Stoph and I waited nervously for the 'dive' before mine to finish, I couldn't help noticing how positive and jolly the atmosphere was. People were smiling, cracking jokes and offering biscuits or words of encouragement as they hobbled about on crutches – such a contrast to the gloomy, silent waiting rooms I had been in. The door to the oxygen chamber swung open. Several very sick children were carried out by their parents. 'Well, that's a few more cancer cells dead, then,' said a mother to her daughter as she pushed her out of the metal dome in a wheelchair.

I was stunned, suddenly humbled by the cheery

strength of this young mother. I was nearing sixty, not in my twenties, as so many breast cancer sufferers are. I had healthy children and we had never had to go through anything more gruelling than the normal slings and arrows of being a parent – one broken arm, one febrile convulsion and a gall bladder operation. I vowed then to try to never feel sorry for myself again. Every time I find myself slipping into that deep well of self-pity, I remind myself of that young mother and her daughter to bring back perspective.

The theory behind hyperbaric oxygen therapy is that you need about twenty sessions in quick succession, and then about one or two treatments a week after that, as kind Jan, who runs the centre, explained as she handed me my own personal mask and told me how to look after it. I booked several sessions in that first week, which also happened to be half-term. As well as several MS sufferers in the chamber on that first afternoon there was also a good-looking boy of about fourteen who thrashed about in his chair as I fumbled trying to put on my mask. His mother sat beside him on a fold-up chair, placing sheets of puzzles and test questions in front of him to keep him occupied.

Christoph peered nervously through the porthole, wondering if I was going to go through with this. I gave him a thumbs-up as the door was sealed shut. The air hissed with oxygen as the volunteer handling the dive began to reduce the pressure. I felt my chest tighten with fear and breathed in deeply. The fresh, pure oxygen felt like sweet nectar. I closed my eyes, trying to calm myself with breathing, in and out, in and out, as my ears popped.

The boy opposite began to moan and wriggle with frustration at being trapped as his mother continually encouraged her son to go back to the board of puzzles on his lap. I couldn't help but admire her patience and her courage. Again and again she kept him on track, focusing him on the worksheets in front of him, telling him off when he thrashed his legs about, or whenever he pulled off his mask and hit her in the face out of frustration. Why were they there, I wondered. They had obviously been dozens of times before, for his mother seemed relaxed and knew what to do, helping me to open the valve on my oxygen supply to increase the flow when I was finding it difficult to breathe.

An hour and a half later, as the dive began to come up slowly, the boy seemed calmer and his mother could turn to her book for a few minutes. As we stumbled out through the tiny door into the bright natural light of day, I asked her where they lived. 'Somerset,' she replied. 'We used to live in London but this is still the closest place for us. Nowhere else will take him – they don't believe it helps for autism.'

'And does it?' I asked.

'Well, I wouldn't be here if it didn't,' she replied with a smile.

Of course. Humbled again by such a stupid question.

By day three of that half-term week the boy was asleep in his chair instead of wriggling about. And after that session he walked calmly to the car by himself, looking just like any other fourteen-year-old.

Oxygen therapy appears to help a whole host of symptoms, from broken bones, wounds, burns and the bends to chronic conditions such as MS and brain damage. With cancer, it helps the chemo to penetrate the cells. It helps ease the pain in my broken ribs and fragile vertebrae, and it helps to beat the cancer back. It takes up a lot of my time, but it's worth it. It doesn't hurt. I can sit there with a book, or meditate as I breathe in deeply, focusing on the in breath of clean, health-giving oxygen and the out breath, where every toxin is sucked away. Phones and tablets have to be on flight mode so I can't work and nobody can reach me. It's a little oasis of peace, surrounded by people handicapped by different conditions, a small community of support.

The oxygen chamber is never dull. I have seen a middle-aged Turkish woman with no English banging angrily on the door during the ten minutes it takes for the dive to be brought up to normal pressure because of her claustrophobia. I have heard a woman complaining about the smell of curry after an Indian father brought out his three-year-old. Another snatched a bottle of face-hydrating mist from my hand as I squirted a few refreshing drops around my nose before putting on the mask with the words 'I'm allergic to perfume' as she sat next to a young woman half her age with a chemo cap on, who looked green and skeletally thin from all the drugs she had to endure. But I have also seen great kindness too – the man with MS who hands out sweets before the start of every session; the young beautiful mother who can barely walk but always cracks a joke or has a funny story to tell. I once sat there while two middle-aged women managed to talk through most of a session, through their masks, about their idle sons.

There is one session, though, that sticks in my mind more than any other because it seemed to encapsulate so much about the fears and the differing doctrines that surround cancer treatment. There were two others in the chamber on that afternoon, a lovely lady with extra-ordinary dreadlocks tied up into a knot on the top of her head, and a small old man with a German accent who looked as if he might have been a Jewish refugee. He seemed highly anxious, and sat rustling a large file of papers. As the door was sealed shut he asked the lady with the dreadlocks whether she had cancer. She nodded. He then asked her if she was on chemo. She said, 'No, I had cancer a long time ago,' and he said, 'Good. Chemo kills. It vill KILL you.'

'Thanks for that,' I interjected. 'I'm on chemo,' and went back to my book. He looked embarrassed but managed to throw pitying glances in my direction throughout the dive, as he handed the lady next to him some of his papers to read, but not me. She would be interested in them; I would not, he presumed, because I had shaken hands with the devil. As the dive came up slowly and we took off our masks, the lady with the dreadlocks asked me kind questions about my cancer. She told me that she had had breast cancer too and that it had gone into her lymph nodes. I then turned to the old man.

'You may think chemo kills, but I know it has saved my life. The question for me now is how to get off it.' The kind lady nodded. The old man shifted uncomfortably in his chair. I wanted to be rude, to say what on earth are *you* worried about? With prostate cancer at your age, something else is bound to kill you first, but restrained myself. Instead I stood up, the first to leave, wished the kind lady a warm goodbye and walked out of the chamber with my head held high. He had no right to judge me, for every cancer in every person is different and the only way we can cope with it is to respect the decisions that we each make as individuals about our treatment.

I thought about that old man all the way home, a little upset, with his words that chemo would kill me ringing in my ears. It's the view of many in the 'alternative' world when it comes to cancer treatment. Chemo destroys white blood cells as well as cancer cells and, with reduced immunity, should the cancer stem cells reignite it can spread quickly because the body lacks enough vim to be able to beat it back. It's a strong argument. But I also know of many people who have survived this brutal, toxic treatment. And I know that it was almost certainly the chemo tablets that saved my life. After the third dose of the first cycle I woke up at 2 a.m. needing a pee and felt suddenly better, different. I could feel this large black cloud drawing back above my head, like opening the sunroof to a car to let in the light. Something had shifted. The same thing happened after taking the third dose of the second cycle and then of the third, only each time the dark cloud was fainter.

It's the polarity of views, the clash of doctrines between the medical world and alternative treatments, that I find unsettling, for there is no one truth, no certainty. At one end of the spectrum there are the dieticians and 'alternative' cancer experts who say that chemotherapy is promoted heavily by Big Pharma, and so profitable there are powerful vested interests to make sure it is prescribed. They say that it can kill people quicker than cancer and that the body has the power to heal itself if you feed it the right foods and supplements, take all of the stress and emotional lows out of your life and detox daily. At the other end of the spectrum is the highly respected medical world, their treatments based on the empirical evidence of peer-reviewed studies and drug trials.

All of the literature and guidance you receive as a cancer patient stresses the importance of making sure that you check with your consultant about anything else that you are taking in case it should interfere with the drugs. At my second meeting with the charming, charismatic oncologist I asked him about diet. 'We have dieticians here. You could talk to them. Changing your diet costs nothing, treating a cancer patient costs, on average, one hundred thousand pounds.' Crikey. Tread carefully ... On my third consultation, when I revealed that I had given up sugar, because the other 'alternative' world believes that cancer feeds and grows on sugar, he said, 'But you need some sugar, and cancer will find it wherever it is in your body from other things that you eat.' Probably, but at least this way I am not making things any easier for the bitch. As I stood up to leave and slipped on my coat, I dropped the news that I was taking a range of supplements (suggested by Patricia Peat to ease the side effects and help build up my immunity) and that I was juicing raw fruit and vegetables daily. 'I presume you don't have a problem with any of that?' I added casually. He nodded and told me to keep going. 'B12 is good for the neuropathy too,' he said, but then I could have sworn I heard him muttering under his breath, 'but it won't do any good.'

I understand that when you see as much death and devastation as an oncologist does, every day of the working week, there is little choice but to be sceptical, to cling to the certainties of science and to be wary of offering false hope. But hope is all that a cancer patient has to cling to in those devastating first weeks and months. Chemotherapy is Big Pharma, but there are also countless other charlatans operating, probably even on Harley Street, who peddle false hope with miracle cures and tonics that are, in all likelihood, useless. We know that conmen excel at being persuasive and believable, particularly when people are so desperate to save their lives they will try anything. But I also know that in spite of the fact that doctors are clearly kind, learned and want the best for their patients, I am just one of thousands who, devastated by this diagnosis, drift in and out of their consulting rooms every year.

The nurses and health practitioners you meet along the way can be economical with the truth, just to get their job done. At my first PET-CT scan I expressed concern about the radiation from the injection of radioactive sugar. Cancer lights up the scanner as it greedily seeks out that sugar. A very pretty Spanish nurse told me not to worry, that there was no more radiation from this than you get on an aeroplane, 'and you don't mind flying, do you? Some people have these scans every week.' So I lay there quietly waiting the requisite hour for the radioactive sugar to circulate around my body before I could be scanned. At my third scan a radiographer, holding the syringe of radioactive sugar so that I could see it, said matter-of-factly, 'You'll be radioactive for about six hours, so stay away from pregnant women and small children until about six thirty.' I burst out laughing. He didn't understand why I should find his cold delivery of such a shocking image so funny. No wonder they leave you alone for an hour and then avoid you as you leave the scanning suite. To them I glowed like a fluorescent light bulb.

The more I read, the more confused I became about such differing theories around treating cancer. So I had no choice but to become the journalist I know how to be, researching every single aspect of alternative therapies and cancer treatments across the world in what has become known in our house as 'Katie's Cancer Hour'. I couldn't take much more than an hour a day of delving deeply into the heart of the beast running rampant through my bones without feeling sick with terror, but hiding behind the ignorance of denial would, I slowly came to understand, be ultimately more damaging. I had to consider every aspect of the multitude of different treatments out there, so that I, and I alone, could decide what might be the right way forward for me, and then live with the consequences. That's a very lonely and terrifying place to be.

I avoid medical statistics. I know how skewed and demoralising they can be. I am an individual, not a statistic, a survivor of past traumas, a freelance warrior. Mercifully my charming and charismatic oncologist (and no I am not in love with him, but I can see why so many cancer patients fall in love with their consultant through the strange intimacy that builds over time, with life and death decisions) has been clever enough not to give me the answer to 'How long have I got?', which I haven't asked for. For how can he really know? He does, however, stress how important quality of life is and the need to balance that with the treatment. If the side effects are too hard to live with, my body needs a break.

His discretion means that I am able to focus only on ways to get better, perhaps even for good. I investigate only what others say has helped them to recover their health. And then I google that vitamin, supplement, treatment with a vaguely scientific name – ARSOTA, a 'non-toxic anti-cancer vaccine'; intravenous high-dose vitamin C; infra-red therapy; bio-oxidative therapy – to consider whether it might be for me.

Certain things came up again and again. Oxygen and infra-red heat treatments seemed to be used in cancer clinics all over the world. Detoxing and reducing inflammation in the body with large amounts of raw fruit and vegetables seemed to be common too. Certain compounds such as Boswellia serrata, turmeric and cannabis oil appear to have anti-cancer properties, as do certain foods such as green tea, berries and broccoli. These were the elements I began to introduce into my daily life alongside the chemo, determined to do everything in my power to live and stay living for as long as possible, just like that old Jew in the hyperbaric oxygen chamber. The urge to survive is the most profound human instinct. Nothing was going to stand in my way when it comes to beating the bitch back for good.

At first, this all felt too 'out there', but it was all there was to cling to. Then slowly, as I grew stronger and looked healthier than I had done in years – even before I was ill – and the side effects of the chemo began to diminish, I began to trust that every single element of my new daily routine of stretching, juicing, supplement-taking, acupuncture, Chinese herbs and deep, meditative breathing was helping me to get better. I bought an alkaline water filter from Germany to take out the chemicals and heavy metals from the numerous litres I drink every day to rehydrate and flush out toxins. I bought an infra-red sauna blanket and lie sweating for forty minutes on days when I am not in the oxygen chamber – another good recommendation from Patricia Peat. It's soothing, relaxing and eases the aches in my ribs. Cancer cells dislike heat while immunity is triggered by it, and some of the toxicity of the three strong drugs circulating through my body is doubtlessly being eliminated through the sweating. I always feel better afterwards: calmer, cleaner, with a clearer mind and far more energy.

I have slowly introduced other things into my daily life which some will consider completely woo-woo. I rub cannabidiol (CBD) balm and frankincense mixed with coconut oil into my breasts and the surrounding area, which is full of lymph nodes. Early research evidence suggests that this ancient essential oil might shrink tumours. Those three wise men may have known more than we can ever understand when they brought it as a gift to the baby Jesus. If bad stuff, compromising our health, can be absorbed through the skin, then why not anti-cancer good stuff too?

I swallow CBD capsules – the non-hallucinogenic, legal

component of cannabis – whenever I feel the slightest anxiety about anything, to take the edge off the fear that I might not have long to live, for I don't need the extra anxiety that comes from that, nor is it good for a body coping with enough stress already from just processing these drugs. At night I take the fully loaded and therefore illegal cannabis oil, complete with tetrahydrocannabinol, to sleep deeply. A tiny drop under the tongue is all it takes to wipe me out. I don't need to wake up at 2 a.m. and lie there terrified, imagining my funeral and whether anybody will be there, or whether the food will be something better than sandwiches or M&S canapés. Please, no canapés. Sometimes when I wake in the middle of the night needing a pee, I realise just how stoned I am beneath the cosh of sleep. I turn on all of the lights and clutch the banister as I walk slowly downstairs to the bathroom so that I don't fall and break my neck. And each time I giggle at the irony. Life has come full circle. I used to crash out stoned almost daily as a teenager to escape unhappiness. Now cannabis fills me with the joyful hope that this ancient medicine might just be keeping me alive. I don't care if the cops come and get me for drugs. In fact, a part of me would like to see them try!

Fighting cancer is like fighting a forest fire. You need an arsenal of weapons at your disposal to beat it back, not just one or two. This is just what I have to do each and every day to feel as good as possible. And I will do everything that I believe might be able to help provided there are also enough hours left in the day to enjoy living the life I have left.

'It's good news,' my oncologist said, almost skipping back to his desk after greeting us at the door to his room for the results of the first PET-CT scan just before Christmas. 'Cancer activity has dropped from 5 to 1.5.' I had no idea what that meant, but it sounded good. The treatment was working. He was pleased for me, but doubtless he was also enjoying personal professional pride in having picked the right combination of drugs. I had no idea then just how lucky I was, for often, particularly with triple negative breast cancer, treatment doesn't work at all.

As he pulled the driver's door shut, Christoph burst into tears of relief, something he very rarely does. 'I thought he was going to say that it had spread,' he cried as he blew his nose. We sat there in the dark of the early evening as the rain began to fall on the windscreen, holding hands in silence, dazzled by the news. In truth, I had always known that the treatment was working. What I hadn't realised was that Christoph was hiding from me his deep fear of expecting the worst. He couldn't feel what I felt as the cancer retreated and he couldn't allow himself to believe me when I tried to tell him.

I texted my brother from the car and he called back immediately, breathless with relief. 'Thank God! Thank God!' he said, as a committed atheist. 'I haven't slept for days.' Texts from daughters and close friends flew back with happy emojis and the warmth of their love. 'Keep doing whatever it is you're doing,' my boss said. And once again I felt loving support raising me high above the ground. But their reactions surprised me more than the scan results. I could see suddenly that all this anxiety and uncertainty about whether I might live or die soon was far harder for them than it was for me. All I had to do was trust that my treatment choices were the right ones. And then commit to them. Friends and family felt powerless.

At the following consultation I asked about the possibility of being put on an immunotherapy trial as this new innovative treatment hasn't yet been licensed for breast cancer. My oncologist shifted uncomfortably in his chair, reluctant to disappoint me. 'There is nothing to measure in the first place because it's only in your bones, so that makes it difficult . . . but if and when your cancer comes back, and we can measure something . . . Then we can think again.' He used the word IF. For the first time he opened the chink of a possibility that I, not the cancer, might win. He has always been so keen to hammer home the certainty that it will return because, of course, in his experience it nearly always does. But that one tiny word, *if*, means that I can dare to dream. With enough determination and focus on putting my health rather than the cancer at the heart of every day, with enough belief that I am stronger than it is – as well as an entire life change with good diet, attitudes and a multitude of different treatments and supplements, then . . . I might just live.

Perhaps all that really matters is belief. That I will go on living in spite of the lows, the rage and the anguish, because without that belief I cannot remain positive, and positivity is, we're told, key to healing. We know that belief is a powerful force. Panaceas work because of belief. Belief is at the root of every religion. Belief is what keeps us going. If we believe, we can. Just as the belief in Father Christmas makes him come in the night to fill stockings with presents, I have to believe that I have the power to heal with the right help. I have to believe that with each supplement, every capecitabine tablet, every deep breath of oxygen, every acupuncture needle, massage and yoga pose, however wacky-woo-woo they might be, I am chipping away at this disease that is a part of me. Healing comes from within as well as from without. We trust our bodies to recover after falls and operations. With enough love and laughter in my life I believe I just might stand a chance of seeing my first grandchild, as well as holding Christoph's hand as he grows frailer and needs me – as I now need him.

After the third PET-CT scan in March, which showed no cancer activity at all ('That's as good as it gets,' according to Patricia Peat), my smart and charismatic oncologist could sense my eagerness to bolt. I hate taking the drugs. I like throwing the last dose away as an act of rebellion when the side effects get too much. Those treated with line chemo rarely do more than six cycles because the body cannot cope with such toxicity for longer, but capecitabine is weaker and so the philosophy is to keep going for as long as I can hack it, or until the cancer comes back. 'What if I go off the drugs, scan regularly and smash it back again with the drugs if it does come back? Wouldn't that be just as effective?' I ask, hoping for a reprieve.

He looked solemn. 'As oncologists, we don't know the answer to that . . . ' Which means this theory hasn't been tested and so there is no empirical, double-blind, peer-reviewed evidence, but at least he is being honest about the limits of our understanding about how best to fight this disease. 'But it feels risky to me. Why change a winning team?' He hammered home the fact that I am living on borrowed time. My cancer would come back. Take a holiday now. It could be three to six months, or longer if I'm lucky. I left his room reeling with the real-isation that if I was to come off the drugs I would have to be the one to make that decision. He wouldn't do that for me. It feels like playing Russian roulette. Is staying on the chemo tablets doing me more harm than good now that the cancer is inactive, shredding my immunity and therefore my own ability to heal? Or is it the key component in the panoply of treatments and radical life changes that seems to be keeping me alive? I can't know the answer to that. Nobody does. But it does feel risky to stop taking them now, when I can just about bear taking them. It could be that not taking the chemo will be like pulling out the one Jenga block that will make the whole tower come tumbling down.

What a stark life-or-death choice. But at least it's an active one that I make about my own well-being. I can't just hand over that decision to an expert, nor should I. Because the most important aspect of every single treatment, every supplement and every morsel of food that passes my lips, is that I have decided to take it because I believe it may help. That sense of agency, of being in control of my own health and doing everything I can to help myself, integrating 'alternative' methods with the conventional medical advice, gives me hope and helps me to accept what has happened. It means I retain my dignity and my sense of autonomy.

We say a great deal about who we are and what we value through our actions and decisions, through the risks we take with our careers, health and lifestyle choices, through our politics and contributions to others, whether we stand up for our beliefs and speak out against injustice, or remain silent. I am not prepared to give in to the disease or trust it entirely to one treatment discipline alone without question. If and when the day comes that I decide to give up chemotherapy, then I will have to live with the consequences. In the meantime, I can only hope that it prolongs my life and my quality of life long enough for something less toxic and more effective to come along.

If we value our freedoms, we have to take responsibility when it comes to freedom of choice, even as we stare deep into the abyss. With every decision in life, whether it is where to live, who to have children with or what career to pursue, we cut off thousands of other paths and possibilities that might have been better. I choose, therefore I am. That's how we feel the power of being alive. With every hard choice we write the script of our own lives rather than sleepwalking through it, at the mercy of fate, or denial. That's the truth I have to cling to now. Because this is about more than just treatment choices; it's about how to choose to live each day and about the dozens of tiny decisions that I have to make about how to get the best out of each hour. It's the very opposite of the passivity that cancer tries to impose as it sucks energy and suffocates life.

It's maybe too easy, I am beginning to think, to just trust that by taking a pill or a course of treatment we can get better, instead of taking a hard look at our lifestyle. Perhaps instead of medical solutions, dismantling the edifice of comforting indulgences – alcohol, sugar, rich food, laziness and stressful busyness – would be more effective. I feel a little stronger each day, from the exercises, the walking, the detoxing and the diet. I tell myself that only one small bit of me has cancer, the rest is healthier, far healthier, than a lot of those I see around me. I have no doubt too that the more I build up that healthy side, my quality of life will improve because I will feel better and my body will be better equipped to fight the cancer. Nobody has the answer. There is no magic bullet. Which means that I am the one who has to become the expert, I have to believe that I can beat this, trust my instincts and listen to what my body is telling me every minute of every day.

The best way to cope with this continual unanswerable quagmire of weighing up the risks and benefits of treatment is to expand my thinking and place it in a wider context. That's all I can do. This is just how it is for most people as we age. We develop painful conditions, which need medication. We take risks with our lives daily, jaywalking across a main road on the phone, skipping a red light in a car, cycling to work through busy traffic. We could slip and fall every time we run up and down the stairs. But we don't think about any of this as potentially life threatening when we are well. Only when we are ill do we see death in every tiny decision.

My oncologist never holds back from stressing that my cancer will come back and he has good reasons for saying so. It must be hard to do that job and stay positive about better outcomes when most patients die. But he did add a caveat at one of our meetings: 'For a small number of people it doesn't come back, but we don't know why that is.' An honest, intelligent answer yet again, for as specialists they can only concentrate on their one narrow field and the patients they see. But Dr Kelly Turner and her Radical Remission Project have collated anecdotal evidence from people who have survived cancer against the odds. She has identified nine common traits: radically changing your diet; taking control of your health; following your intuition; using herbs and supplements; releasing suppressed emotions; increasing positive emotions; embracing social support; deepening spiritual connection; and having strong reasons to live. I think I at least stand a chance of fitting into that small category of people whom my charming oncologist cannot understand. I like that. An outsider. A rebel to the end.

'Oh oncologists *always* say it could come back in three to six months,' Patricia Peat told me on the phone when I relayed our conversation after the first all-clear scan. 'Stay off the sugar, and keep pummelling it with oxygen and heat, and it won't come back.' She sounded very certain and entirely positive about that.

'Really?'

'Really.'

It's not a hard decision choosing who to believe – his narrower view based on science or her woollier, wider one. Peat's belief cannot be based on peer-reviewed studies or large-scale trials because they haven't been conducted. She has to trust the evidence she has seen with her own eyes, but that's good enough for me. Likewise, Radical Remission's conclusions may not be 'scientific' but they are based on extensive interviews with real cancer patients – exactly the same methods of investigation I have used for my own books on family life. I trust my own findings, so why not trust these too? It's scientific enough for me.

Time will tell whether the charming oncologist or the positive Peat was right. One of them will be. But in the meantime, as I adopt all of these new practices, there is also the slow dawning of a new reality, which hits everybody in mid-life. Whether it is cancer or some other more minor ailment, ageing well has to be about taking charge of your own health. With my new routines I am beginning to feel better and happier than I can remember feeling in a long time.

i am a cancer warrior

I start each day with some geriatric yoga – a hesitant shadow of what my body used to be able to manage. In classes I was always, without a doubt, the least flexible person in the room, but every time I walked home feeling taller, calmer and encouraged by my slow, incremental progress in some of the poses. The effects seemed to last for days. I know that it is through yoga that I will regain some of the muscle strength I used to have before this dramatic, sudden weight loss. And it is yoga that helps me to focus on what really matters at the start of every single day.

Chemo clouds the mornings. The side effects are always worst when I wake up. They build up overnight in a resting body. Slowly, consciousness rises from the cosh of numerous drugs, and then the stark truth dawns: I still have cancer. I burrow deeper under the duvet and want to stay there. Why bother to wake up? Why bother to go through yet another day filled with so many hopeful anti-cancer activities if I only have months or just a year or two to live? I lie wallowing in the deep, warm oblivion of sleep until a cup of green tea is lovingly brought upstairs by Christoph.

I unroll the yoga mat and stand tall. I raise my arms high above my head and think of some of the many things that I have to be grateful for. For the rich life I have lived and the life I have left, for all the loving support I enjoy. Then there is my body and the amazing work it's doing to try to heal itself. I thank my doctors, who are all exceptional in their fields. I am lucky not to be going through this alone. I feel nothing but gratitude for the treatments and the fact that there is some good news to be found in all this darkness. I do not need surgery and the cancer is in my bones, not my vital organs. I thank Stoke Newington – for my neighbours, for the park I can walk to, for the wealth of local shops, for the fact that Whole Foods and a plethora of organic, juice-able vege-tables and essential anti-cancer supplements is less than a hundred yards from my front door. We practically live there. Usually there is much more to be thankful for than I have time to list before my arms start to ache and I have to drop them.

But it's exhausting. The prospect of the hours ahead spent fulfilling so many tiny acts of self-care – oiling my dehydrating body, swallowing supplements, juicing, exercise, lying under the sauna blanket, resting my aching back, deep breathing – feels pointless. Almost every other day there is some treatment to get to – hyperbaric oxygen, acupuncture, massage or the Chinese herbalist. The time invested in looking after myself now comes close to a full-time job. Sometimes I think it would be a good idea to put everything onto a spreadsheet so that I don't have to remember it all, but there never seems to be the time. Occasionally I don't feel grateful and I sob instead, when nobody can see me, my face buried into the yoga bolster I used to be able to lie back over with such ease to stretch out my back and chest muscles. I drown in the emotions of bereavement: from denial and rage to despair. I cry for the loss of the future I had always imagined I would have. Then, when the sobbing dies down, I dry my face. Stand up, stand tall and start the day again, for there is no other choice.

I stretch the aching muscles of my sides and my back, inserting space between each crumbling vertebrae with care. I spread the soles of my feet wide, rooting them to the ground with my body weight to try to ease out the pain of nerve damage from the chemo. Come back to life, feet! Don't leave me more compromised than I already am. Then I work tentatively at the muscles of each leg, opening the joints of my hips and lifting my thighs in a gentle march.

It is only when you get this sick that you realise how precious the strength in your legs is. Bending down to reach for something, climbing stairs, getting into a car are easy, subconscious acts until you have three cracked ribs and enough cancer coursing through your bones to light you up like a Christmas tree on a PET-CT scan.

As my body stretches slowly into life and the beginning of a brand-new day, a fresh optimism begins to flood through me. I feel grateful for the years I spent attending gruelling weekly yoga classes, where the mats smelled of sweat and other people's feet. I was terrible at backbends, and whenever the teacher asked at the beginning of the class who had their period, I always put up my hand so that I could get out of doing terrifying headstands. (Yogis believe a menstruating woman must keep her hips low to help the drainage of blood.) But those weekly classes have taught me how to focus all of my attention inwards. I know how to press every square millimetre of each palm flat into the mat as I throw my weight forward, or backwards into the tips of my toes; I know how to ease out my sacrum so that my fragile spine has a better chance of supporting me through the day. And I know how to breathe into the back of my lungs, imagining every tiny molecule of oxygen pushing away any thought that the cancer in my ribs may be invading further, and then exhaling long and hard, washing everything bad away.

When I drop into warrior pose, pulling my arms taut and wide, I begin a morning battle mantra. *I am a warrior and nobody fucks with me. Especially not cancer.* I imagine myself plunging a large samurai sword into the dark, evil, blobby matter of cancer and then hacking it into small pieces. Then I see myself hoovering up every last shred of the disease. For some weird reason, in my imagination, the black bits are scattered about like pieces of torn paper on a sanded wooden floor, when in fact our house is carpeted throughout. And then I carry the Hoovers down the front steps. Our smiley postman with dreadlocks is always there, standing at the top of the steps as I open the door. 'Let me help you,' he says as he takes my Hoovers and then helps me to hurl them one by one into the rubbish van. We stand together and wave goodbye to them happily as the wide jaws crunch and swallow them whole while reversing out of our tiny cul-de-sac. We seem to be getting through a lot of vacuum cleaners. But that's cancer swept out of our house for another day.

Sometimes in my daydream I insert sound effects for extra vim: a rageful sigh as I plunge the sword deep into the heart of the beast, the hum of the Hoover, the sound of my feet on the concrete steps or the rubbish van's *Beeb-beeb. Vehicle is reversing. Please take care.* And sometimes my mind wanders further away, to thoughts of food and anti-cancer recipes I could make, which I take as a good sign. I might be getting better.

I can feel the side effects of chemo easing as my body gets going. This way I get to stay on top of it before it demoralises me too much and diminishes any hope of being able to live a normal life again. Chemo dehydrates, so after yoga I squirt drops into my dry eyes, facial oil into my nostrils, which minimises the nosebleeds. Chemo can crack the soles of the feet and the delicate skin around the nails, rendering a person with compromised immunity highly vulnerable to an infection, which could kill quicker than the cancer. So I rub special serums around my nails and massage a mushroom-based cream into my soles – one which has been developed specifically by an innovative Spanish company.

I get dressed slowly and carefully go downstairs. Everything has to be done mindfully, with the focused fluidity of a tai chi practitioner so that nothing is jerked or damaged, so that I do not hurt myself by slipping, juddering my spine, or falling over. I take care so that I do not cut myself with the knife as I chop up fruit and vegetables for the NutriBullet. At the breakfast table the pill-taking begins: probiotics to ease the gut, CBD for the pain and a concentrated mushroom supplement to help boost immunity. Then it's the first juice of the day – three or four different fruits and vegetables pulped with kefir to line my gut, topped with a teaspoon of Cordyceps powder, turmeric and one pod of frozen live wheatgrass – followed by a healthy breakfast of berries, more kefir, almond milk and a little muesli chewed slowly to stop the nausea swelling. Then yet more supplements – Boswellia serrata (frankincense), giant bone-support calcium pills that are almost impossible to swallow, grapeseed extract and kelp, washed down with another cup of green tea. And then it's the chemo. Five pills followed by yet more pain relief in the form of a cocktail of Tramadol and paracetamol.

It takes me about an hour and a half now just to get up in the right way, in my way, so no more breakfast meetings. And that's just the morning. If I were to add up all the hours I spend building up an anti-cancer body it must take up to half of each day, every day. But if that's what it takes to choose life over death, then so be it. I've never been a high-maintenance woman, putting on a face of make-up every morning, visiting hairdressers weekly for a wash and blow-dry or a manicurist for my nails, but now seems like a good time to start to take care of my body. But instead of moving from the beautician to the podiatrist, I visit the hyperbaric oxygen chamber, the acupuncturist, the masseuse, a Chinese herbalist. It is only by attending to every single tiny and seemingly trivial aspect of this new regime of self-care that I can escape the sense of being trapped within a desperate helplessness that would leave me languishing in bed for most of the morning. But it feels odd somehow, incongruous with the patterns of the past, where a working mother always has to put herself last, not first.

Mothers are lay psychologists, therapists, teachers, chauffeurs, playmates, nutritionists and story-readers. Most of us want to be able to do all of these things because otherwise what on earth is the point of being a mother? But that means there is never enough time for the luxury of doing just one thing at a time, for considered slowness or an empty stillness to focus.

I have been so busy juggling work, motherhood, shopping and cooking over the past twenty-five years that doing everything with speed seems to have changed me at a cellular level. I rushed rather than strolled. I found it hard to do anything slowly, easily irritated by those who seemed to think they have all the time in the world. Because I am a left-hander in a right-handed world and played the piano throughout my childhood, both my hands are almost equally strong, making multi-tasking easier – I can stir a simmering white sauce to stop it from going lumpy at the same time as chopping up the steamed cauliflower to go into it with the other. My mind was always full of lists and responsibilities, and racing from regular hits of caffeine.

I knew that losing my independence by giving up work to look after the children full time would be disastrous personally and compromising for our marriage and our standard of living. I don't regret a single aspect of that decision and the health and stability of my adult daughters is testament to the fact that it was the right thing to do. But it's the racy speed of everything. It's the way my life seems to have sped by so quickly because of all that busyness. It's the lingering regret that I didn't feel able to slow down and relish those fragile moments of time.

With grown-up children the need to rush around has

slowly lessened. There was more time for me. For us. But even then I was so programmed to cram as much as I can into every day that relaxing into an armchair and staring out of the window, thinking of nothing at all, felt alien and wasteful. But now, with cancer stepping so neatly into that empty, available space, I have no choice. I have to prioritise my own health for the first time in my life. I can only do one thing carefully at a time.

While the rest of the working world seems to spin faster and faster away from me, I eat slowly, one mouthful chewed over and over again rather than gobbled greedily as I used to do. I walk gingerly, giving everyone I pass a wide berth in case they bump into me or are riddled with a contagious infection. I concentrate on the pills I have to take with each meal so that I take the right ones, and all of them, for there are so many to remember. I work at my job and then rest in between tasks, telling myself that doing nothing with my eyes shut each day, focusing only on my slow, deep breathing, will fortify my immune system a little more. One social engagement or outing a day is enough. And if I am to go out in the evening, I nap in the afternoon. I have to, just to be able to relish the joy that comes from going out to supper with friends, to a concert or the theatre.

When you're well it's easy to take on too much, flattered by the fact that you're apparently indispensible, terrified of saying no in case that means being less well thought of or overlooked next time. But when you're severely compromised physically, you have no choice but to give priority to what matters. And that means shedding every unenjoyable, time-wasting or stressful duty. Do I want to go to a publishing party for a book I haven't read and an author I've never met, or have dinner cooked for me by my daughter? No contest. I can say no to invitations, work or people who drain my precious strength with a clear conscience. Pacing my energy through each day is all that matters, so that I can take pride in being able to walk a little further, climb a hill or laugh at full throttle the way I used to, a laugh so sudden and loud that it has been known to make sleeping babies cry, without fearing pain as my ribs begin to heal. Being with those I love and with nourishing activity is what matters now. There is really nothing else.

A large shining light is to be found in slowing down, in focusing only on getting well and in thinking about what one has in life – even when the diagnosis is shit. When you stop rushing around you notice the tiniest details, the sensuous impact of ordinary beauty: the dark lushness of a blackberry, the burst of its flavour in your mouth; the bright glimmer of low winter sunlight through bare trees; the clear pure sound of a barn owl twit-twooing in the dark quiet of countryside deep in the night; the tingling touch of Christoph's hand in mine; the gentle tenderness of feeling like young lovers again because that one point of intimate connection feels as intense as a first kiss. Every moment feels brighter, more precious and more alive because I know, really know now, that it is all so very painfully temporary.

Yoga helps to slow everything down and steady the mind. By focusing inwards, all that nerve-shredding outside noise has less volume. Yoga helps to silence all those ruminating, pernicious thoughts that feel so negative; it soothes anxieties about not doing anything productive in a day, or about a future I cannot predict. Yoga first thing in the morning isn't a source of spiritual sustenance. I do not need a religion to console me with life after death. But it offers a lifeline, helping to focus on nothing but my one small and imperfect body, switching off stress hormones and slowing my breathing. Nothing out there matters more as I start the day, this precious day, other than the miraculous feel of fresh air in my lungs, the strength of my legs holding me up, the feeling of space between my ribs as I hold my head high. There is no room to think about anything else as I relish the liberating feeling of a taut muscle easing as it lengthens a little. Perhaps this is spiritual in its own small way, for closing one's eyes and focusing down into one's own steady beating heart is, after all, at the root of prayer.

Yoga helps too with the problem of denial. I was so certain that I didn't have cancer through all those early tests in the autumn of 2016. It was osteoporosis. Just broken ribs. There had been a mistake. Then I found it hard to believe that this was an 'advanced' cancer, an 'aggressive' one that I couldn't beat. I still don't. I even wonder sometimes whether the diagnosis of triple negative could be wrong, for back then my oncologist answered my questions about the tests' accuracy with the startling statistic that there was a one in twenty chance that it wasn't triple negative, which seems quite high to me.

Denial can be useful for coping. It blinkers the mind, helping us to forget past traumas or avoid dealing with current problems. Denial helps us get through. If I look the other way, if I say again and again that this can't be true then maybe it won't be. But shutting the mind down in this way can also stifle the ability to adapt to a new reality. I know this. I saw this countless times as a mediator. And yet now, when I must adjust to my own new reality – that I may not have long to live – I feel the clouding consolation of denial. Reality is too painful to contemplate for long.

I suspect, grudgingly, that a sense of acceptance is what I need, more than anything, in order to be able to cope. The rational part of me knows that if I accepted this new reality, life would be easier. There would be more room in my mind for healing strategies and more energy for living each day to the full. I know I need to let this happen, and yoga helps.

Over the years I have learned to recognise and then accept the limits of my body as I try to stretch into that perfect reverse triangle demonstrated by the teacher and cannot, or wobble precariously on one leg as I stretch up into tree pose. I have had to learn how to foster a relaxed ease, opening up my body rather than forcing it into different positions. Even though I haven't been to a class since all of this cancer malarkey began, when my forehead touches the mat in child's pose I can hear my old teacher telling us that this calms the mind, and it does. Suddenly there is a blissful nothingness in my head. Not one thought. With yoga practice there is no other option but to become rooted in the moment, as I focus only on spreading my toes and rooting my feet into the mat.

And with a regular routine and daily repetition of certain poses I can sense the smallest physical improvements as I stretch higher or feel the ligaments opening a little more in the back of my knees. With daily repetition my body seems to absorb stillness and I can measure how, slowly, my strength seems to be building up again. My arms are becoming strong enough to hold my upper body up into a plank now, when previously I couldn't lift a large book. The joy when I could stretch into a dog pose again and push my hips high into the air gave me a smile for most of the morning. This meant I was getting better. This was progress.

Yoga and my other rituals make me aware of something else: the repetition of all these poses and body-care regimes has become addictive. I follow the same routine every morning. It helps me to remember everything, but it also means that if I run out of something like broccoli sprouts or kefir I am thrown. I recognise that there is now a rigidity to the structure of the day, which is close to obsessive. The more out of control you feel about your own life, the more addictive these rituals become, and I know that I have an addictive personality. When I lived close to a swimming pool and used to swim several times a week, just walking past the local baths and smelling the chlorine made me want to go in.

Nine months after the diagnosis, I have moved a little further away from complete denial and accept the idea that I am dealing with something very powerful and dangerous. I find myself going back over the pictures on my phone. It helps me to look at how ill I used to be, so that I can monitor how much better I am now.

There's a picture from Devon, our first weekend away together. We stayed in a wonderful country hotel with good food and rolling grounds. But I could only walk hesitantly down the drive and back again because of the pain. I remember how frightening the dining room felt because it was packed with people sneezing with streaming colds. That was then. Now I don't think twice about walking for over an hour or eating out in crowded restaurants. That's progress.

I notice that time takes on a different dimension when you are this ill. It slows to a crawl and yet paradoxically speeds up at the same time. The date at the top of each photograph on my phone reminds me how recent all that incapacity was. It was January then, at that country hotel. Now it's just June and I feel so much better. I remember seven years ago, when my book *Couples* was published, Christoph did an interview with a journalist about what it was like to be married to a 'marriage expert'. She was quite taken with him and described him as 'a stylish, charismatic character with state-of-the-art glasses ...' I had it printed on a T-shirt for him, and on the back, another quote: 'You can't imagine women don't throw themselves at him and apparently they have.' He was so embarrassed that he would only wear it in bed, but it made us laugh every time he did. Now I notice the date at the bottom of the quote: 2010. It feels like such a long time ago. Another era entirely. That's consoling too, for maybe, just maybe, in another seven years' time I will look back at this year and feel it to be equally distant.

Acceptance helps to clear the head. It creates mental room for more important things such as asking the right questions and living each day to the full. Acceptance allows perspective to widen. If I helicopter up above myself I can see this whole experience as simply part of getting older rather than solely my own narrow grief. Something was going to get me eventually – arthritis, diabetes, heart disease, emphysema. I could have had an accident that compromised my life with pain, mental illness, depression or disability years ago, but I didn't and that feels lucky. I marvel at mothers giving everything they can to their disabled children and am grateful that we were spared that. I stop and watch people in wheelchairs pushing themselves along the road and wonder how much that must hurt their arms. I see people muttering, unkempt and smelly, and wonder what life must have done to them to push them so far over the edge and feel grateful that life has never been that bad for me. So maybe even tussling with the toxicity of chemo is part and parcel of growing older. For if it wasn't these drugs it could have been others. So many people my age are on different types of life-saving medication with side effects. This is something I am learning slowly to accept. And taking these life-saving drugs is, let's face it, better than the alternative.

Slowing down is integral to growing older. Maybe, as I approach sixty, it was time, even if I had escaped illness, to ease up on that brisk pace. Focusing on that helps me to accept my own limitations now. The new normal. What's hard, galling even, is that I am so much more aware of a clamouring to fill my days with a million joyful pursuits in case I never get to do them again. It is painfully ironic that, just as I have come to really understand how limited time is, I lack the stamina to achieve more than one or two things a day, and with plenty of rest in between. I have no choice but to appreciate the minutiae of each day as I move through it like a snail. But maybe that too is just a more extreme version of getting older.

I know now that there is no point in getting het up in a traffic jam or manoeuvring through endless lane-jumping on a motorway in a misguided attempt to get ahead like I used to do, to gain an extra minute or two of time – even if my life expectancy is shortened. Better to still the mind with deep breathing, picturing the beach hut, or listen to something soothing on the radio. I used to get so anxious if I was late or hadn't achieved much in a day. Now it couldn't matter less if something on my very short to-do list doesn't get ticked off. There is always tomorrow. And the next day. Just maybe not the day after that.

Better to have an afternoon nap when I feel my eyelids drop rather than struggling on; better to go to a very special concert because the music will be nourishing and uplifting, even if that means sleeping late the next day; better to sit talking with either of my daughters about their lives, imparting whatever wisdom I may have, rather than working. I now resist the urge to fill every hour with enough 'constructive' and distracting busying activity as possible.

Acceptance brings release. Cancer has brought to an end my compulsive need to achieve and prove my worth. I could see cancer as a guillotine that has come down between my life before and my life now, but cancer also feels like a bridge between these two very different worlds. I am walking across it from a life full of competitive ambition and thrusting-about-town-ness, to a slower, more contemplative pace. I am putting my health and my needs first each and every day, possibly for the first time in my life. It helps to remind myself, in that first yoga pose of the day as I reach my arms up to the sky, how rich my life has been so far. Focusing on everything I have had helps me to forget everything I might lose in the near future. I am slowly learning how to be well through being this ill.

Then we went in for what we thought would be a routine, scan-looks-good meeting with the charming oncologist. 'Bones are fine, but there's a question mark over your liver,' he said. First thought: fuck. Second: I don't believe it. 'I have my doubts that this is cancer, but it could be.' So we went for an MRI – the best way of seeing what's really going on in the liver, a notoriously shy organ when it comes to scanning.

All of the anxieties of last autumn came tumbling back in the days before we got the results. I couldn't eat or sleep properly. My liver began to hurt badly, suggesting that there could be something wrong. I got the runs. And a million different thoughts flew through my mind, from denial – *I'm fine, the imaging is wrong* – to petrifying fear – *what if it isn't?* I felt a burning sense of injustice – *it would be so unlucky to have only three months cancer free, given that I have worked so hard to try to beat it* – as well as an understandable weakening of my resolve – *why bother with any of this anti-cancer stuff if it doesn't actually work?*

But I didn't collapse, signalling perhaps that I had begun to accept the new status quo. I didn't gobble an entire packet of chocolate digestives as I might have before this diagnosis, because I know refined sugar compromises the immune system as well as feeding cancer. I think I might be well over the bridge between denial and the acceptance of cancer as my new lifelong companion.

At this scan I didn't experience the same sense of categoric denial as I had when I was first diagnosed; now it was more a sense of resignation. If it was cancer rearing its ugly head again, I knew, calmly, that I had no choice but to accept it, because of everything we have been through in these past nine months. I would take a deep breath and then consider, what now? I feel my resilience growing. I am stronger and less terrified of dying than I was nine months ago. If it was a secondary cancer in my liver I would just have to cope, and find ways to redouble my efforts when it comes to fighting this disease.

In those harrowing hours and days I realised something else: uncertainty is the name of this game. That cancer is always just one sliver of time away from me. I have to be rigorous. Each and every day. I cannot slip with just one pudding, one glass of red wine, skip treatments or walking just because I can't be bothered. I have to accept that this is what life is going to be like for me now – moving from scan to scan, rollercoasting from the lows of *what if . . . ?* to the highs of *it isn't . . .* There will be progress, but there could also be setbacks.

It was good news this time. Cysts on the liver, not tumours. As he closed the door to the consultant's room Christoph said, 'I think this cancer is going to kill me before it gets you.' I laughed all the way down the stairs to the reception desk. However hard this is for me, it is harder for him, holding everything in so as not to make me even more anxious. We were lucky this time. But I think I have finally, if reluctantly, recognised that there could be less good news at some time in the future.

But is this new reality so very different from anyone else's as we grow older? Cancer is preparing me for ageing, increasing physical problems and death. It's also teaching me that I can't control what happens to me, but I can control how I react to it. It has helped me to acknowledge that cancer will now always walk by my side. And I have less fear of the future.

I am just one of countless people forced by illness to accept that I have limited energy and patience sooner than I would have liked. But in the widening spaces, opening up between all these anti-cancer activities, when there is no need to rush just to be able to get through everything I had to achieve each day, there is a glorious sense of freedom, of empty space. The mind can wander back over the past and then think about nothing more taxing than what I might like for lunch.

home

When I found the Denby plates and bowls, the crockery
I had eaten from almost every day as a child, the full
significance of clearing my mother's flat after her sudden
death dawned. We were packing up our childhood as well
as her home. We didn't have much time. The landlord
wanted to take back possession. I thought we had finished
deciding what to keep, bin or try to sell until I opened a
kitchen cupboard and there they were, exquisite subtle
pale grey-blue inside, surrounded by a rich, dark brown.

I was being super-efficient, stemming grief with the
practicalities. There was so much to do: organising pro-
bate, going through my mother's papers and books. So
much of the contents of her flat were just things, most
of them ugly or redundant. An ancient iron. A Hoover.
Mountains of prescription drugs. Clothes and handbags
that nobody in the family could possibly want. Then I

found the bowls and knew I really wanted them. The shape of one of those bowls in my hands felt so familiar that the tears began to flow, finally. I used to slurp cereal from them every morning before heading to the bus stop and school. I used to wash or dry them every night with my brother. We used to sit in front of them at the black-and-white mosaic table my parents had made from a kit for supper. It was a narrow diet in today's terms – roast chicken and spaghetti Bolognese, a delicious dish of chicory wrapped in bacon and white sauce. Arctic roll or Angel Delight for pudding. I scooped them up and took them home.

Now I eat porridge, or muesli laced with berries and apple compote, from them almost every morning. They sit alongside all of the other crockery I have accumulated and cherished over the years. For I love bowls – large and expansive ones for salads, small and delicate ones for dips, soup or olives. My grandmother was a talented potter and remnants of her creativity sit decoratively on shelves in the sitting room. When my daughters were small I took them to a café called Art for Fun. They painted mugs and plates, some tiles which we've set into the wall above the sink, and a teapot with a happy picture of our family showing no features on our faces other than smiles. We use these idiosyncratic and creative pieces. They bring sunlight into the day with their innocence, with their memories; four generations of family pottery all in one house. My family. My home.

My mother lived in her rented flat for over fifty years
and everything remained in exactly the same place. A
tiny gold-plated inkwell always stood on the windowsill
of the sitting room. The same lamp illuminated the sheet
music on the piano where I practised scales and pieces
every day. The pictures hanging on the walls were never
moved around. The same red wooden chair sat by the
telephone in the hall. I cannot remember my mother ever
sleeping in anything but the single bed with the white
cast-iron headboard, or keeping her clothes neatly folded
in anything other than the giant dark wood chest.

The installation of central heating and the end of electric fires revolutionised her life. For years we had shivered
through much of the winter in thick woolly jumpers that
she knitted in a range of colours. She simply added a few
extra rows each year as we grew. We were trained never
to leave heaters or lights on because of the high costs of
electricity. I still turn off lights as I leave a room.

Eva, my mother, was frugal. She had to be as a single
mother and a professional writer without the security of a
regular job or alimony to rely on as my father often didn't
pay up on time. Mornings in the school holidays were
dominated by the need for silence so that she could work,
but the weekends were freer. I have some happy memories
of Saturday-morning trips to the library to choose a book
for the weekend, the three of us reading the Sunday news-
papers in her bed, and then cutting them up for collages
on rainy afternoons. But mostly my memories of that flat,

my childhood home from the age of five, after the divorce, until seventeen, when I left after a blazing row with my mother, are not good. As I grew older, harsh words began to fly between us as we each tried to undermine or humiliate the other. I had the energy and passion of youth on my side. She had the wisdom, the clever, searing articulacy of a prose poet writer. She usually won, forcing me to retreat to my bedroom crying tears of rage.

When I left I knew I would never go back to live in that flat. I would rather have slept under the arches at Charing Cross than spend another night there. I did return to visit her, though, dutifully each week. But I could never stay for long in this mausoleum, where everything was exactly the same as it had been in my childhood, before I felt the same hostilities between us swimming to the surface, when we both demanded more love and attention than we could ever give each other.

My mother's home had been snatched from her in 1939. So much had been snatched from her at the very young age of seven. Security being the foremost. I came to understand that as I grew up, and how so much of that residual unhappiness tumbled down onto me, her daughter, just as my grandmother vented hers on my mother. Eva found it hard to allow me to flourish in ways that had been denied to her. She was, after all, from that generation of women who had far less choice than we do now. 'You're so much luckier than I ever was,' she would so often say, and I heard it as her telling me it was somehow my fault. As I left that top-floor flat after each short visit, the front door to the house closing behind me with a familiar click, and looked up at the kitchen window where she stood, barely visible above the giant pot of basil that she never seemed to use and we waved goodbye to each other, I would breathe in the sweet air of freedom and then drive away, usually at high speed.

I did all those things that good daughters are supposed to do for their mothers – calling regularly, dropping by, inviting her over for Sunday lunch. But I always kept her at a distance emotionally, boxing her into a separate space simply because she could hurt me like nobody else. Her snide comments, solipsism and all that difficulty between us seemed to linger, the rage of having felt so unloved as a child close to the surface – for both of us. The arrival of my first child and her first grandchild softened things a little. Christoph rooted and separated us with his sanity. He appreciated her intellectual vigour and liked her, but he also understood her power to wound me. 'I've been so lucky with my son-in-law,' she once said, a silence lingering on, implying that, without him, who knows where we would be. As a teenager and in my twenties I was adamant that I would never have children because I didn't want to put them through the same sort of experiences. But then I met Christoph, knew that he would be a good father and that I personally needed to break the pattern, so that my girls could grow up happier and more secure than I had been.

My books helped me too. Decades of research into psychology and the dynamics of family life explained so much about what had happened to my mother as a child and then to me. That new understanding helped me to put some of that history to rest. Eva expressed pride when my books were well received, but never read them. Eva was interested whenever we tried to talk about our relationship and why it might have gone wrong. I explained why her mother might have been the way she was – almost an orphan, who lost her own mother in childbirth and was then packed off to school by her 'wicked' stepmother. I could see a flicker of understanding in her eyes sometimes, but it was too hard for her to change and I understood that. How could she wipe the slate clean if that also meant looking back with regret?

My family and my brother's became home for her as she softened with age and became more vulnerable. We had four wonderful daughters between us and they loved her; her quirks as an old lady were funny and endearing. The balance of power shifted between us. She needed me, us, more. Now that I am roughly the same age as she was in my most vivid adult memories of her, now that I am home-based and vulnerable just as she was, the similarities between us feel uncanny. I see her bony, angular face surrounded by wispy, thinning hair in the mirror, now that I have lost all that 'blubber' – her favourite word for my tendency to be chubby like my father – because of the chemo. I do not see my face, but Eva, in front of me and I shudder. I feel my eyelids dropping at 9.30 in front of the TV just as hers used to do. I think hard about whether I really need to go out if it's raining. She would never go anywhere when it was wet unless you were prepared to pick her up, and then take her home again. I found her stubbornness exasperating then; now I feel much the same way.

There's a creepy circularity to growing older that seems to take us straight back to childhood. Having to go to bed early. Not having the strength to open a jar by yourself. Not being able to reach high shelves any more. Crowds feel threatening. Then because you had to clutch on to someone's hand so as not to get lost in a sea of legs; now because everyone moves so fast and with such determination they could knock you over as they blast past, head down, looking into a phone. Healthy adults seem to dominate everything outside. They rule supreme, while children and the frail have to somehow skulk along the sides, invisible and secondary.

Home is where both the young and the old need to feel safe. Every square inch is reassuringly familiar. I remember tiny secret places in my mother's flat, the few square inches of wall behind the chest on the upstairs landing with a scribbled picture nobody knew about; the book behind which I hid a precious tiny wooden doll so that it would never get lost or stolen. Venturing further than school, the park or grandparents was an outing rather than the daily norm. The world outside was examined from the safety of our top-floor windows: the slow crawl of traffic down the hill in the morning rush hour, and then back up the hill at the end of the working day; the fireworks exploding in the sky on the night before my birthday. My father's home was very different, always changing as he built new cupboards and bookshelves or set about redecorating and rearranging a room. It was always a good place to run to, for loving conversations, support from him as to how to deal best with my mother, whenever life at home got too much.

In the early days of the cancer diagnosis the home that Christoph and I have made became a welcome sanctuary, unthreatening and familiar, the place where I felt protected, fed and cosseted by the love of those around me. My bed, womblike with familiar comfort, was the only place guaranteed to offer the release of deep sleep. Everything I needed, painkillers, chemo, the right anti-cancer foods, teas and supplements, had its place, within easy reach, and the idea of trying to go somewhere without these props felt impossible.

Christoph's need for displacement activities during my illness means that he has at last fixed everything that has been irritating us for years: the magnolia in the garden is finally freed from the clematis that has been strangling it; the kitchen chairs no longer wobble; useless or broken utensils have been thrown away. Some repairs to the most basic of home functions became more acute because of my vulnerability. The loo seat always wobbled. When my frame was healthy it never bothered me. Now, every time I sat down it slid about beneath my bum and shafts of pain travelled up my spine. It was even agony if I had to bend to put the loo seat down after Christoph had used it. Blame erupted, punctuated by humour: 'I've been trained as a boy to lift the seat. It's going to take time to train me to lower it as well.' But he then called in a handyman to fix the seat.

Once again this narrow Victorian terraced house that has been our home for thirty years has been reconfigured; every stage of family life has demanded a different use of living space. At first we needed a changing table, stair gates and a highchair. Then all that had to go to make way for toy cupboards and pop-up Wendy houses. Buggies made way for bicycles, tennis rackets, Rollerblades and skateboards in the hall. The kitchen table became our parliament, for discussion of family matters at supper every night and a place to do homework together.

Now the top drawer of the old toy chest has been cleared for my drugs; the infra-red sauna blanket now lies on the spare bed for my daily sweat. Christoph is here most of the time, doing all of the washing, shopping and cooking, so he has reorganised the tiny cupboard where the washing machine and dryer live. For decades I used to have to twist into contortions getting the washing into the dryer and never thought it could be any different. No longer. For he has swapped the appliances around. Simple. Why didn't I think of that years ago?

My treatment takes place at home too. Every few weeks a nurse arrives to take my blood, check my temperature and blood pressure. If the bloods are OK the following day is set aside for treatment. We take over the sitting room and I lie on the sofa dozing, surrounded by books, framed photographs of my babies, and my grandmother's pots. Clare attaches the drip and does her paperwork over a cup of coffee while the Avastin drip-drips down the tube into my arm. I like Clare because she has a sense of humour. And I like the feeling of home wrapping me up in its familiar care as poison floods through my body.

As a young mother, I used to dream of escape, of a more expansive layout with far fewer stairs and different views from the windows. It felt depressing to think that this might be the last place that I would live. Since I am freelance, I have made this home my workplace too. My life is all wrapped up here. Now, the idea that we might ever have to move, or downsize, feels like the worst possible outcome, for this is where three decades of precious memories lie, embedded into every chipped cup, every chair, every inch of grubby paintwork and floor. Some of the curtains are ragged or bleached by the sun, skirting boards are scuffed, the kitchen could really do with a coat of paint, but I don't care any more because these are the markers of a home well used. I once dreamt of stripping out the bathroom, which was installed before we moved in. I used to gaze longingly at plush bathrooms with free-standing baths and elegant tiles all the way up the walls. But now, every time I lie in a hot bath and stare up at the picture of our old dog, I can drift back to nightly bath-times, to mountains of bubbles and splashing laughter and remember how that dog would sit waiting patiently for the girls to get out so that he could lick the sweet soapy water off their legs.

Memories fill the void caused by the boredom of convalescence. The entirety of the happiest years of my life is trapped within the air here, and I can breathe it in, smell the mess of life with small children as I relish the peace of solitude now without them. To lose a single memory would be heartbreaking. I can lie in bed and spool back to delicious lovemaking, or sleeping babies between us and Christmas mornings opening stockings.

I can lie on the sofa and see my daughters playing on the floor with their Groovy Girls, Polly Pockets and a range of Sylvanian Families on board their red and green canal boat. The art cupboard in the corner is still full of the paints, pads of paper, coloured card, boxes of beads and sequins that they used to pull out once their homework was done. We covered the kitchen table with newspaper and spent countless happy hours painting or simply making a mess. At Christmastime we sat here smothering cards and labels with glitter and glue. And the food. Oh, the food we used to eat off this very table. Fish chowder was one of their favourites. Roast chicken and an aubergine pasta sauce, all cooked in the same pots that we still use today, and eaten from the same plates and bowls that now hold the food I force myself to eat so that I can swallow five pills of chemo as well as all the supplements.

Sometimes I think I can hear the girls running around upstairs or rowing, one accusing the other of stealing their clothes. As I pass the rooms they used to sleep in, where the unwanted stocking presents still linger, and old stuff that they didn't want enough to take with them but can't bring themselves to take to the charity shop either, I see them. There are the books I used to read to them at night, the old soft toys that comforted them. In the garden, that precious tiny square of greenery and fresh air that gets no sun at all from early December until the end of February, I see them hosing each other down on sweltering hot days or searching for the place where their father once buried their dead hamster in an empty teabag box. And mysteriously, every summer, a Red Admiral hovers about the flowers in exactly the same place where we released the ones they had hatched in their butterfly farm nearly twenty years ago. The label on the box they hatched from said that might happen. Perhaps just as salmon leap up rivers and waterfalls to spawn where they themselves were born, just as swallows fly northwards for hundreds of miles over the Sahara without ever stopping just so that they can lay their eggs in the same place every year, we all need to return to some place that feels like home.

I grow stronger and more able to venture out, and everything from the GP surgery to pharmacies to Whole Foods is within easy walking distance and so familiar I feel a possessive, proud ownership of the place where I live. That's home too. I used to take the children to the park, and stood bored and cold in the playground while they scampered about with sheer exhilaration. I took the dog for walks there while they were at school. I played tennis there. Now I walk around my home patch gingerly, stretching strength into my legs, breathing in deeply, and stare in wonder at every new budding flower and blossoming tree as if I am really seeing them all for the first time, because this could also be the last time I see spring.

Abney Park Cemetery backs on to the end of our street and when I am at my most angry and despairing I stomp and cry there. Why does it have to be in my bones, why does it have to be triple negative and not some other sort of cancer? The dead that surround me are consoling. They seem to say, you will be fine. No point stressing over the inevitable. And then happy memories of past times in that lush, wild Victorian cemetery come flooding back. Running with the girls down paths to the large stone lion that sits on top of a tomb so that I can lift them up to ride on his back. Visits every Christmas morning to see if Santa has dropped something extra for them as his sleigh flew over our house – an annual tradition to get them out and into some fresh air for a while. He always did. They would squeal with delight as they found a small wrapped-up present beneath the shrubbery, or perched on the edge of a grave. And then that astonishing promenade production of *A Midsummer Night's Dream* that my daughter Eleanor, now an actor, had always dreamed of, and made happen, at the height of midsummer. We queued up patiently at the main gate after the cemetery was shut and were led by fairies to various key spots for sections of the play: decorated covens for Titania's bed, long paths for the young lovers to lose one another on. As the light dropped we were surrounded by magic, by the herbs and flowers that Puck uses to make merry mayhem and by the sparkle of lights hanging from the trees. Each time I walk past the place where Bottom sleeps with Titania, or the ruined chapel where we sat on logs to watch the final act by the mechanicals, I smile and remember. I feel pride swell at her achievement and am no longer sad.

I can only cope with the stress of cancer by trying to get rid of all the other stressors of life and it is being home that helps the most with that. I can turn the outside world off. I can avoid the telephone or the front door. Being at home, surrounded by all this familiarity, provides the scaffold to recovery. Without that central plank, everything else feels much more threatening and destabilising. It is the mundane ordinariness of domesticity that is so reassuring, the mindlessness of washing up or wiping down the kitchen table exactly as I have always done. It is the familiar sounds of people going up and down the stairs, the feel of age-old mugs in my palm, the instinctive knowledge in the middle of the night of exactly how many stairs there are between bed and bathroom. It is being able to throw tantrums of distraught rage and self-pity, kicking the walls with sobbing histrionics – 'I am too young to die'; 'It's not fair' – in private, free from prying, judgemental eyes.

When I first walked into this house, heavily pregnant, I knew immediately that this was where we would live. I could even see where the Christmas tree would go. And there is has stood every year. This year, the first with cancer, I knew that Christmas had to be exactly as it has always been for us as a family. Every ritual had to be the same, from the stockings at the end of their beds, opened all together on ours, to the book stacks at the bottom of an over-decorated, kitschy tree. Every year since the girls were tiny I have made a careful selection of books and wrapped each one individually in brightly coloured tissue paper, piling them up: the largest at the bottom, the smallest at the top, tied up with a giant ribbon. They love them and always leave them until last to open together. I knew that this Christmas, more than any other, we had to maintain that continuity of tradition for our girls. This time I wanted to give them something enduring and special. Their empty stockings changed magically overnight into expensive leather weekend holdalls stuffed with presents. These bags, I hope, will accompany them on their travels through life, and each time they will take a little bit of us with them too.

When it came to putting up the Christmas tree, Grace and her boyfriend took charge, with me directing from the sofa, propped up by cushions. Understandably, as this *is* such an important job tension grew. While her boyfriend relished the pleasure of positioning each fairy light perfectly on a real tree, for he had only ever had plastic ones as a child, Grace began to get agitated. Suddenly she burst into tears and it all spilled out. This wasn't going to be a happy Christmas like all the others had been. The stability of her world had been rocked to the core by my illness. We hugged, all three of us. And for the first time since I had been diagnosed, I took charge as a mother should. I reminded her that I had no intention of dying any time soon. I insisted this would be just as happy as all the other Christmases have been. We cried, and then we hung every single bauble, all the swinging plastic glittery Cinderella slippers, woolly dachshunds and gaudy Arsenal paraphernalia we have collected over the years on the tree, before pinning the smiley, shiny fairy she made at nursery school on the top.

The Bechstein baby grand piano was the last object to leave my mother's flat. It was the only item named for me in her will. I used to play it daily and loved to lose myself in swirling, all-absorbing tunes and the sheer concentration of making two hands do very different things at the same time. That piano symbolised home for me. My mother died believing it to be her most valuable possession, and gave it to me, unaware that the cracked soundboard and frame meant that it required complete reconditioning.

I thought long and hard about fixing and keeping it. That piano had meant so much to me. The tone was beautiful and my fingers were able to fly up and down the keyboard with ease, for each key seemed miraculously to descend with exactly the same pressure. But it would require an entire room and we simply didn't have one going spare. It was sentimentality that made me want to keep it. I no longer play and have found it impossible to take it up again because I can no longer give Chopin preludes, Bach's two-part inventions and Schubert impromptus the technique and musicality they deserve.

Eva's flat was empty of everything but that piano. As I waited for the specialist removers to come I ran my fingers up and down in a chromatic scale. I played 'Chopsticks', loudly like I used to do because it irritated my mother so much. It was a precious musical instrument for proper music, she would say, not a toy to be bashed at. The emptiness of the rooms, devoid of pictures, furniture and all the knick-knacks I have looked at all my life, hammered home the truth that all of this was now finally, really over. My mother, that difficult, demanding, wickedly bright and verbally dextrous woman who had dominated so much of my life, was dead. She would never come back. I would never come back here, to the place of my childhood. And then I sobbed loudly against the music stand until the piercing sound of the downstairs buzzer announced the arrival of the removal van and brought me back to practicalities once again.

It was the dismantling of that flat, which had always been home, however unhappy I had been there, that catapulted me into middle age. My childhood was ancient history and now, with both parents gone, I was next in line. But here I am, just five years later, facing that possibility and doing everything I can to fight it. Eva found it hard to accept the frailties and indignities of ageing. When she was at her most angry she would say 'Just you wait until you're older, you won't like it one little bit.' And I'd tell her that I'd find my own way of dealing with it. Now here I am living with infirmity and toxic medication, trying not to be as difficult and demanding as she was, and probably failing.

Grief lingers. It washes up suddenly like a great wave, knocking you over with unexpected force. I miss her, as I miss my father. Their power is great: they seem to hover around me. I hear their voices. I see their faces in mine. I laugh as I imagine what they might say or think about Brexit, Trump or the colour of a new jumper. That's the power I will leave behind too, the essence of having been really known. It will pervade every piece of crockery I have eaten off, every bowl I have tossed salad in, every chair I have sat on, the tapestry cushion I made when recovering from a miscarriage, a small token signifying that lost child, and the bed that I lie in, staring out at the changing leaves of the silver birch trees on the street outside, with a mug of tea held to my chest.

My overwhelming feeling at Eva's death was one of relief that she could no longer hurt me. I would no longer have to feel guilty about her unhappiness and all of the things she demanded of me that I felt unable to give. My parents did their best. They knew no better. I may see my mother in the mirror at times, rather than my own face, but that means I also have the best of her – a refusal to be typecast, an ability to speak my mind, a strong sense of values and morality, an occasional twinkling wickedness in the eye. I hope to improve on my technique for this as I age, as she did.

But when a parent with whom you have had a difficult relationship dies, that grief feels compounded, complicated by all the losses. I felt as if I had lost both of my parents twice. My father's death from cancer brought back the loss I felt when he left me when I was a child; my mother's brought back all that loss of the missing love that I felt I had never had from her as a child. And so they haunt me more, perhaps, than parental ghosts do for others who were happier as children.

The last conversation I had with my mother was on the telephone, just before I went on holiday with two girlfriends. 'You mean Stoph isn't coming with you? How wonderful.' She was genuinely thrilled that I might have some man-free time. She was always a feminist, right through to the end. But it was the new tone to her voice that surprised me. She wasn't resentful or envious of the fact that I was travelling when she could not. She wished me *bon voyage* and I believe she really meant it. This, I realised after she died while I was on that holiday, was the best parting present she could have given me, last, heartfelt words of warmth and tenderness – the way I had always wanted them to be between us.

The home that the four of us have made here in Stoke Newington resonates with mess, love and laughter. It's a happy home, full of people coming and going, and there is always enough food for a sudden surprise visitor. This is my home now. My real home. The longer we live here, the longer the walls absorb the changing dynamics of family relationships as we all grow older and have to deal with whatever life chucks at us, the more that unhappy childhood home recedes into a distant memory, now that it has gone for good. This home, my home, seems able to contain the worst of us, sheltering us from the outside world by bringing out the best in us.

Getting so ill, and so suddenly, inevitably strains family life. Christoph has had to learn how to multi-task, and that isn't an easy thing to learn in your sixties. We used to divide the chores up – he sorted the rubbish and did all the washing-up, and as a hands-on, loving dad took responsibility for looking after the girls' eyes and teeth, making the appointments and then booking time off work to take them. I was home for the girls while he worked and I did all the shopping and cooking. Now he insists on doing everything, and even though I see the strain, the bags beneath his eyes, he never snaps or complains. I try not to complain either when something isn't as tasty or cooked in the way I would have liked, just as he rarely complained when I was the one doing all the cooking.

We have managed to come together and redefine our roles as a family. We are no longer the two powerful adults, determining the lives of our children. We are four autonomous adults, equal in our standing within this house as they come and go frequently and do what they can to help – showing us how to work apps on our phones or find Netflix on the remote. I know that one day, possibly even quite soon, all that could change, should my health deteriorate even further and our nuclear family reduce to three, but with this confidence in the strength of our home I know that they will cope, and that I will live on for them in this house.

The girls move in and out regularly because renting anything in London eats up so much of their low incomes. In the spaces between them being here, Christoph and I have found an even deeper intimacy as just the two of us. He now understands more of how my life was when the children were small because he is now a carer. I read while he cooks, when it used to be the other way around. Occasionally, when we cook together, creating what we would like to eat in the kitchen that has nourished us all for so many years, chatting about everything and nothing, I feel so close to him it is as if there is no air between us and we are joined as soulmates from shoulder to hip. Held by him within our home. In those calm moments, when our daughters' anxieties are not here to mingle with ours and we have no idea what they are up to, there is a very special kind of peace, where we are allowed to be older together.

Cancer has brought us closer as a family: it has highlighted the spaces between us as well as the uniqueness of the bonds that will always be there. The quality of our relationships is so much richer, more intimate and honest. But particularly for Christoph and me, this feels like a very precious and special place to be. Every hug, every morning spent drinking tea together in the bed that we have always slept in, every fond memory or story shared, even though we have both heard them dozens of times before, unites us in this life we have made for ourselves, in this loving home we have created and value above anything else.

from loss to less

Mid-life houses loss. There is so much to mourn. Loss of youth, beauty and sexual allure as heads no longer turn. Flirtation is rare and feeling desired is now a thing of the ancient past. There is loss of energy, evidenced when the prospect of going to bed at 8.30 with a book and a hot chocolate is more enticing than going out to a party. Loss of deep, uninterrupted sleep, and instead lying awake at 3 a.m. listening to the black silence of night or the World Service, wondering whether you will ever get to sleep straight through the night again, appears to be common as we age. There is the loss of young babies and children who have become grown-ups. There are the lost names of people I have met, books read, films seen and places visited. There is loss of friends and family, either to death or to distance – they simply live too far away to see. And then there's the loss of idealism or hope that things might ever change for the better as a new cynicism about the intransigence of inequality takes hold, a realisation that politics seems incapable of fixing injustice.

Cancer has magnified mid-life angst a zillion times over, an accelerated form of ageing. I have been catapulted into feeling old before I am. The slow loss of sex appeal associated with an ageing woman – that feeling that you could go out with a paper bag on your head and nobody would notice – has speeded up. I haven't lost my hair, so am not obviously a cancer patient, but strangers seems to stare through me and those who know me cannot help but look at me with sadness in their eyes. The skin on my stomach is suddenly wrinkled and saggy because of the weight loss and my bottom seems to have disappeared completely. (Let me know if you find it.) In the early days of great pain from the cracked ribs, I longed to be touched, to feel the connection of intimacy, to feel less isolated in my affliction and to lose my sadness in the exhilarating sexual release of feel-good hormones. But, terrified of more pain, I needed a cordon sanitaire of about a yard all around me, and Christoph was understandably frightened of coming close. He too felt the stress of my illness and the burden of caring; it shut him down, just so that he could cope.

Opportunities and ambition are suddenly more limited. Some are amazed that I am still working. But work is a large part of life, so refusing to relinquish my place in the world of work really matters. It's sad to think that I might never write another book, but that merely makes me all the more determined to make this one a cracker. The idea of achieving anything new in my career is laughable, which makes me want to do the job that I have even better. What grows through all this loss is a new enthusiasm for staying alive and living the best life possible. That feels more ambitious than anything I have ever attempted or achieved before.

Psychologists talk about reframing the negative to find something more positive, and never have I needed that technique more than now, for there is so much new loss to contend with. I have lost that innocent certainty I used to have about living a long and healthy life. I have lost faith in my body, for it has let me down. I have lost the belief that you can recover from illness, for even though I feel better and scans suggest that cancer appears to be beaten for now, it will always stalk me from the wings. And I find it hard sometimes to trust my own mind because of 'chemo brain' – a fog that descends when the body is too toxic. I lose keys, forget the point of conversations, and can be late for appointments, if I remember them at all. I am beginning to resemble a dotty old lady.

It helps to think of all this not so much as a time of great loss, but of needing less. There's a new light to be found in this profound life change, for I am often happier now than I have ever been, which feels like cancer's final ironic twist.

There may not be a far future for me, but that means less to worry about. No point dwelling on whether I might get dementia or be unable to pay for my care. I used to worry about ending up a bag lady, wandering the streets and going through people's rubbish looking for things to keep me warm, a relic no doubt from my Jewish past when our family lost almost everything. Now my pitiful pension prospects because of a life of self-employment no longer bother me.

As a control freak it is scary to see how cancer has so easily sucked away my need to be in charge. In the early days I couldn't shop or cook and lost control of my ultimate female powerhouse – the kitchen. I set up an account for online shopping and then several days later, lying on the sofa, I heard Christoph and Grace in our basement kitchen, trying to figure out my password so that they could order things. 'Try Kate57,' he said. Smart. Obviously a weak password – name plus year of birth – since it took them no time at all to get into my account. 'You're in? Great. Now what do we need?' Absolute silence. They had no idea because they rarely did this sort of regular shopping. The kitchen and what we eat were my domain. They didn't have years of experience walking around the supermarket, knowing exactly where eggs, cream or pasta could be found, or what might be picked up usefully for the next meal. I had a list of essentials in my head every time I went. And so I lay upstairs, in pain, barely able to move, with that list running through my head, imagining my habitual trek up and down the aisles. 'Tinned tomatoes, loo paper, eggs ...' I tried to shout, but felt so weak my voice wouldn't carry. On they struggled, trying to think of something to buy on my credit card. 'I know!' exclaimed Grace. 'Dentastix.'

'Great, get ten packets,' Stoph replied. I sighed. At least the dog would be happy. And then the confirmation email came through on my phone: a long list of all sorts of things we really didn't need, and certainly couldn't eat.

Budgeting has gone out of the window. If I need supplements, organic fruit and vegetables, Chinese herbs or expensive lotions I find myself buying them. I buy clothes too. All that previous questioning – Do I really need this? Will it make me look fat? Do I have something already just like this? Do I deserve this? – has gone.

I operate on short-term planning and give into immediate desires: I get good seats at the theatre or the opera and couldn't care less about parking tickets or speeding fines. And instead of worrying how to get around London and topping up my Oyster card, I drive or take taxis, never risking infection on the Tube, in case I should end up on intravenous antibiotics in A&E. All of this may be flagrant, but to my mind it seems a good use of the money I earn.

I find I worry less about those I love. I haven't the energy or the clarity of mind to try to help them when they are unhappy or troubled by something. They will have to take care of themselves. It's liberating to feel less responsibility for others, less guilt for failing to do things in the right way. I used to want to make things better for them. There is also no point raging at the failings of friends and family, even the dead ones. I try only to think about what's best about them because that makes *me* feel better.

There is less ego, for the shifts of ageing in the body reveal our true fragility. I may never achieve everything I wanted for myself, but rather than mourning that as a loss it would be better to accept that there is less of a need to achieve, or to be someone out there in the world. And that's liberating.

There is less need to talk or to win an argument. So many things are inexplicable or not within my control as I retreat from the world. If others are boring on about their own views, I let them, preserving my own energy when I used to want to talk all the time. I worry less about what other people think of me, what will happen to the earth, about politics or the state of the nation. And I couldn't care less now about never getting that wraparound to expand our kitchen into something more bourgeois.

I need less excitement in my day and avoid the adrenalin kick of nail-biting thrillers and dramas. We need less stuff as we age and at times I feel overwhelming urges to clear out anything I no longer like or use. I don't want to be surrounded by clutter. I don't want to see ugly things.

I only want what I love and covet around me. I want to wear clothes that make me look good, look at objects that remind me of the richness of the life I have lived and eat the simplest delicacy rather than mountains of food. Small rebellions thrill me more than ever before, like dumping the last dose of chemo when the side effects have become too much or speeding through traffic lights as they turn red. I am in control of my life and my treatment. This is my life to live as I choose. Nothing more frightening than death can ever get me.

I worry less about my general health too. High cholesterol? Not bothered. Heart attack because of the chemo? Well, at least that would be a quick way to go. The one consoling thing is that I do not look as if I have the Big C. Everyone tells me how well I look. Ten years younger, they say, bolstering my self-esteem. So that's all right then. At least I don't have to worry about that.

I remember the strangely prescient philosophy I developed to cope with the seismic changes and losses of mid-life before I was diagnosed. Every time a decision had to be made I would ask myself what I would do if I had eighteen months to live. Would I spend the afternoon visiting that person, would I see that play, do this ironing? When friends talked about dilemmas in their own lives, I would sometimes ask them the same question.

I knew that the answers would probably be different if you really did have only eighteen months to live. But now that I could be in that position I see that's not so. Would I be disappointed if I died never having been to Australia? Not really. But that would have been the case whether or not I have cancer. Doesn't that philosophy make you more selfish, a friend once asked me. Why should it? I would spend an evening watching the daughter of a good friend in a dreadful play if I thought it would help show support with or without a shortened life expectancy. Knowing that I want to do all those things I enjoyed before, living a good life, my life, without a bucket list of extraordinary adventures is enough.

With every tear I shed I feel as if some deep bubble of sadness has been punctured, gone for good. There is less and less to grieve as time goes on and I regain aspects of my former life. I need less. I find I need fresh air, a beautiful view, nature and the arts, which resonate with the significance of life and loss, so much more than I ever used to.

Good storytelling, music and drama freeze time and soothe the soul with the common tragedies of humanity. They calm my anxieties by focusing only on the present. Past and future disappear. The collective experience of listening to live music is meditative. Every strand of a swirling orchestral piece, every note of an aria, feels grounding as the notes pin down each moment in time. Sitting still and listening can make entire hours pass without the thought – Help, I have cancer – ever running through my mind. I need less variety too. Anything by

Bach is almost enough. Everything is there in his master-ful scores from searing sadness to soaring joy.

This year I have read eleven works of historical fiction, one after the other, and then read them again as a judge for the Walter Scott Prize for Historical Fiction. It isn't a genre I have voluntarily read much of before. But in those pages I found a deep mine of consolation. They placed my experience into a wider context. They made me feel lucky to be alive today, rather than in times before anti-biotics or pain relief. People have lived through famine, war, poverty, and lived a far shorter, less rich life than I have. They have suffered destitution without support from the state. I just have to get through cancer at a time when new, successful forms or treatment could be on the horizon.

It helps too to feel wrapped up by nature, rooting my feet on uneven ground, breathing in the sweet scent of leaves, grass and pollen. Walking through any landscape reminds me of the relentless circularity of life.

In spite of so much loss to ageing there does seem to be one final gain. The differences between the sexes seem to diminish as oestrogen in women and testosterone in men dwindles. With my illness, Stoph has stepped into the caring role I used to occupy. He is better at ironing his T-shirts than I ever was. He takes pride in the way the kitchen is always spick and span and I never feel that sighing resentment of having to clear up after others *again*. We share the cooking as I teach him how to make risotto or chicken soup and he develops the confidence to experiment with new recipes. We lie in bed together each morning drinking tea, with Zeus nestled between us, as we look out at the silver birch trees shimmering in the wind outside, watching them grow slowly green with fresh leaves and then brown with the autumn. We laugh over the silliest things, sharing memories of our children and each other. We hold hands and are kind to each other.

I may have lost the future I imagined for myself but I have each day, and that makes me want to seek out the best of it, with Christoph, my magic man, by my side. There is such joy to be found in the deliciousness of the ordinary. Lying in the warmth of bed with our legs entwined while the wind howls outside. The joy of being able to lie on my side without pain as my ribs mend means that I can hug him in the night and then go back to sleep, spooning. I can do more than just hold his hand for comfort. I can breathe in the scent of his neck again and savour the feeling of flesh against flesh, or the softness of the cotton sheet beneath us. Every tiny detail feels so poignant and so very precious.

Just being alive is enough for me now. And it is such a wonderful life. With so many memories of far busier times, I don't need anything more. And it's perverse, that just by doing less, wanting less and mourning less there seems to be so much more time in every day for anything that can make a good day great – a delicious flat white from a pavement café watching all the people go by, the sound of the wind rustling through leafy trees, a really good book. There is time to reflect and for small, less ambitious plans – learning some German, perhaps, or picking up playing the piano again. The losses of middle age may feel huge, but the gains are great too and I can feel myself stepping up into that new way of life with surprising ease.

endings

At the end of Year One on Planet Cancer this is what I know: that the difference between me and someone seemingly without cancer is a compromised immune system, that cancer thrives on sugar and doesn't like heat or oxygen, that the Big C never really goes away, that getting on top of it involves a paradigm shift in every aspect of your life – a colonic irrigation of mind, body and soul – and that you can never go back to the carefree days you had before, where death hovered faintly on a distant horizon. Only I didn't think that my life was that carefree then, not until cancer came along and showed me what I had before.

I never knew that three of the ugliest words in the English language – zero cancer activity – could sound so beautiful after six months of treatment. I never knew that I would hear the word protocol almost daily. It's not a word that I'd ever heard much before. But on Planet Cancer, it governs everything from the strict rules around highly dangerous drugs to the process for admitting patients on chemotherapy into A&E. There are individual protocols too, new bespoke daily routines around all the other ways that you can help to beat the cancer back, from juicing and supplements to massage and cannabis oil. Because cancer is like a forest fire raging and destroying everything in its path it takes an entire arsenal of heavy weapons to dampen it down and put it out.

After three clear scans I am cautiously growing more confident about saying 'I am recovering from cancer', even that 'my cancer is dead'. The clinical term is inactive, implying that it could always rise up again. It lies dormant in my bones, a sleeping dragon. And so I tiptoe around it, swinging between two extremes – gloomy thoughts of time being so limited that I should just eat anything I want every day of the week and spend extravagantly on luxurious treats, to saving everything I have for potentially life-saving treatments. I know I have to stay positive, for the mind controls everything. I understand that I have to keep on battering it with good food, supplements, exercise, positivity, detoxification, a stress-free life as well as buckets of love and hugs from all those around me, all day every day, to make sure that the tiniest new spark is killed before it can reignite the tinder box of my vulnerable body. I'd like to live so long that the insurance pays out more than we've paid in and I become one of those wonder stories that people like to tell when trying to reassure someone who has just been diagnosed with this disease. *She beat metastasised cancer when everybody predicted that she would die.*

I understand that cancer spreading to the bones is not good because that's when it is more likely to kill quickly. But I like to think a little differently. Is cancer ever curable? Doesn't it always lurk threateningly once it has struck? I still like to believe that I am no different from anybody else who has been diagnosed with a cancer that isn't aggressive or advanced. If this disease can swoop out of nowhere, like a bird of prey, then it can leave just as easily too.

My year with cancer is slowly turning into a narrative that I tell, rather than one that I inhabit. In September the shock of the diagnosis launched me high into outer space. I sat far away on Planet Cancer, going from test to test, from one doctor's appointment to another, looking back at Earth with everything I knew or understood spinning further and further away from my reach. Now I feel as if I am slowly coming back down to land. My land. A more familiar land as the daily anti-cancer work I have to do becomes routine and I regain much of the life I used to take for granted.

I have given up the intravenous Avastin because a 'systematic review of Avastin and capecitabine in inactive cancer' did not throw up much in the way of conclusive evidence that it would extend my life. I hated taking it more than the chemo. How brave of me, I thought, to finally be able to look at the research and read the data. The major side effects of the drug can be devastating and I was beginning to show evidence of the minor ones. My consultant looked at me sympathetically as I told him I wanted to give it up. I had been expecting a fight. Instead, he simply nodded and said 'I'm OK with that provided that you don't look back and say I should never have given it up, if the cancer comes back, say at your next scan.' An intelligent reply. As we grow to know and trust each other we can be more honest with each other too. I admire his intellectual breadth and his uncanny ability to say exactly what I need to hear at every visit, even if it isn't something I want to hear.

With every new muscle ache, every stabbing pain in my ribs or twinge in my breast, I do of course worry that this is the Big C coming back. Only a nutter in complete denial wouldn't. But several hours can pass now without ever thinking once about cancer. I now view it as a life-threatening condition, which has to be managed but is not necessarily a death sentence. I could easily die of something else first. I hear myself telling someone that I have *had* cancer, and smile at such a Freudian slip. I tell another, a complete stranger, in an email that I am recovering from breast cancer and cannot possibly meet her for breakfast because it takes me an hour and a half to get up and hit send without a moment's regret. I am more able to calm myself with deep breathing or a CBD pill when anxiety about being in such acute pain surfaces. I tell cancer to shut up and get back into its hole and leave me alone. I am not ready to give in to it yet.

As I get stronger I can imagine a time when I might have the confidence to explore and go further out into the world, far from a hospital or even a mobile phone signal that could connect me to the twenty-four-hour service at Healthcare at Home. And I understand now why some people diagnosed with cancer train for marathon bike rides, swim across oceans or take themselves off to the deepest rural parts of South America. It's a kind of healing, telling yourself that you are still vibrantly alive and capable. But I can only look forward with faint optimism because I can also see that there could come a time when I might lose that will to live, because of the pain, because of the exhaustion, because of the lack of a life worth living. But I am not there yet. It helps, though, at the end of this long year to be able to look forward to such a time not with fear but as a welcome release, a blessing, a reversion to some natural order, which is bigger than all of us.

By going to the lows and staring deep into the abyss I can soar up to the highs again and find more reasons to live, as well as the competitive determination to win. So every morning, as I strike a pose, warrior pose, decimating the dark matter of cancer with my imaginary samurai sword, I visualise it as something outside my body rather than some dark internal force that threatens to swamp me. The smiley Rasta postman arrives in real life with a bundle of Jiffy-bagged books. He knows I have cancer. 'Are we winning?' he asks, with no idea that I am using him to help me beat this demon mentally every morning. 'We are,' I reply, and thank him for bringing me the post.

Endings are rarely happy, and I have always found endings hard. I did not like saying goodbye to my father every time he dropped me home. I found it hard to leave jobs or boyfriends in case I should never get another one ever again. The only way I could manage the end of a good holiday was to imagine coming back to wherever we were. I mourned the end of every stage as my children grew up, the end of the intimacy of breastfeeding, the pudginess of their limbs as toddlers, their gazelle-like bodies as teenagers. I clung on to my favourite Babygros, those OshKosh stripy dungarees and that heavenly white cotton skirt flecked with tiny embroidered yellow spots that Grace wore almost every day for two whole summers.

But endings also offer the chance of new beginnings and nothing in my life so far has taught me as much about how to start again as this disease, just as I turn sixty.

There is life before and after cancer. I can never go back to the life I had before. But then that's true of every major life change, isn't it? One stage, such as being single, ends and another, of coupledom, begins. As a new parent I needed time to adjust because everything felt so profoundly different. I was shaken to the core by the suddenness of so much change to my sense of self and my relationships to friends, family and work. I felt I had lost my independence, physically chained to the house, trapped and exhausted by the new routines of infant care. But then I fell in love, really in love with a passion more powerful than anything I have ever felt for any lover, with the tiny, perfect baby in my arms and I never wanted to let her go. Being launched onto Planet Cancer feels equally life-changing, but in the opposite direction. Instead of marvelling at the creation of new life, I have been forced to accept the emotional truth of being mortal.

Before the diagnosis I used to kid myself with the intellectual truism that we all die and that I could cope with that, but these were just words. I never fully understood them. Now that this first year on Planet Cancer is coming to an end, I think I may have finally accepted the ultimate ending of death. If it is cancer that gets me, so be it. Dying doesn't scare me quite so much any more. Perhaps that's because I have lived through the blackest, bleakest despair. But that deep darkness began to fade as my health and strength returned. I have been given a second chance at brilliant, beautiful life and I intend to live it and soar back up to the light again.

It's been a year of extremes. The worst of times highlights the wonder of the best. So many things have come to an end. I have learned how to let go of my children and relish the freedom of not needing to cook or sort things out for them with an absolute lack of guilt. It's the end of the family dynamic we once knew. Instead, two powerful, Amazonian young women, utterly independent, charismatic and capable, stand before us. I am proud of their resilience and how easily they seem to have managed the giant shift in the balance of power with their parents that usually only happens once children become parents themselves. They have grown up because of my illness. Both now see us as older and more vulnerable. They can smell the possibility of my not being around and all those normal mother-daughter tensions have dissolved. We simply want to enjoy each other's company while we can.

Ironically, just as this year on Planet Cancer draws to a close, our daughters have moved back home and we are a four again. This time both are clear that this will be the last time that they will live at home and I am OK with that. This time, though, as their mess mingles with ours and the house feels crowded again, I don't mind one little bit. I smile as I see their piles of clothes shed on the bathroom floor when they have had a bath, their shoes littering the landings and their bikes in the hall, even though they make it almost impossible to get into the house with anything wider than a plastic bag. This is the stuff of happy family life for one last time. Why feel irritated by these minute and trivial things now, when they are so close? It feels like a real ending this time, and therefore I can enjoy them being here that much more.

Christoph has decided to give up work. He has a small pension, the mortgage is paid off and I will carry on earning for as long as I can. That's an ending too. I used to worry so much whenever he threatened to jack it all in. How would we manage without his income? Would he become an alcoholic? How would we manage being together all the time? Now I just love the constancy of his presence. He finds it hard to work and to care for me at the same time, and says that all he wants to do now is look after me. I am touched, flattered and grateful for such a remarkable display of selflessness. He is adamant that my health comes first and that we are in this together. In sickness and in health. Until death do us part. We will spend these last few months and years enjoying a more peaceful time together.

Occasionally extreme emotions surface. I see him sitting next to an attractive single woman at a dinner party and can suddenly see them together after I am gone. Jealousy bubbles up, as does deep alienation and a sense of aloneness. These are emotions that have to be suppressed, however understandable they may be.

I have finally learned how to be at peace with all of the negativity that pervaded the past like a cancer. I want to embrace every last hope that life has to offer me now. The impact of my parents' divorce was profound and damaging. Training as a mediator revealed how deep that damage still was. But those feelings of worthlessness have melted away as I feel love from those around me, more than I ever knew was possible.

endings

Life on Planet Cancer means the ending of fantastical notions of a distant future where we might be richer, more successful or live in some other better place. It is the end of complacency, that naive optimism that things can and will always be this good. It is the sudden ending of the pretence of youth. I can no longer kid myself that I might one day climb Kilimanjaro or visit the Galapagos Islands. Cancer has forced me to accept that I have entered the final stage of life sooner than I would have liked, and suddenly I notice keenly the age at which people have died in obituaries and on tombstones. I watch how the elderly move so carefully and admire their outspoken honesty. It's the eccentrics, the interesting craggy characters with a wicked sparkle in their eyes and kindness in their souls I will model myself on. In spite of all the physical pain from the side effects of such toxic drugs, I will enjoy the carefree release of being rebellious in the months and hopefully years I have left.

It's the end of hours of competitive tennis and the beginning of a more gentle approach to the game. No more diving for difficult balls or running around the court. I have to slow it all down and rely more on technique, but that would have happened anyway as I got older. It's the end of driving solo at high speed to the beach hut in the Mini with the roof down, and the beginning of a new phase where Stoph and I go there together and sit side by side with our books in front of the view. It's the end of lazing around in the sun for hours without any kind of UV protection. My olive skin used to just turn brown in an hour like a roast chicken. Now, with chemo changing everything at a cellular level, I need factor 50.

It's the end of saving clothes for best and the beginning of looking my best each and every day. It's the end of putting off until tomorrow what I can say or do today. It's the end of self-consciousness for I now talk openly to anyone who wants to listen about how I have cancer. It's the end of thinking of time in terms of years, seasons or hours. Instead, it's am I on or off chemo? The months are measured by scans and the days are punctuated by the taking of supplements and Chinese herbs, by the new routines of juicing.

It's the end of travelling light. No more slinging a couple of tops and clean knickers into a bag and onto the back seat of the car. No more freedom of flying with only hand luggage. Now there are bags and bags – one for drugs and supplements, antibiotics and a thermometer in case I should get an infection, another for the NutriBullet, fresh organic fruit and veg as well as a small teapot for the Fortnum & Mason's green tea I need every morning to wake up and quash the nausea. The orthopaedic pillow has to come too, as does the foot massager and the long snakelike hot-water bottle to ease my back pain. I am deeply attached to my pink yoga mat, so that I can start each and every day wherever I am on the right footing. All this comes with us whenever we go away, even for just the night. It's like going back to when the children were young, when packing felt like a military operation and took most of a day to make sure that nothing essential was left behind.

There can never be an end to that deep sensitivity to persecution that comes from being Jewish, with a mother who fled Nazi Germany with her family. Some things cut too deep. That trauma pervades every sinew of our being as a family and can never be exorcised. But its power grows weaker with time and with every generation, and so I have decided in this tumultuous year to find a concrete way to feel more reconciled with such a past. After the Brexit vote in June 2016 my brother and I mulled over the idea of reclaiming our German nationality – a statement of our Europeanism. Then, when I got ill, we decided to apply together. I was born in this country and feel sort of British. Sort of, because being Jewish tends to make you feel like an outsider wherever you are. Germany was the seat of evil for me as a child, and yet it was also somehow a part of me, and my heritage too. I was always suspicious, and never wanted to go to Germany. Whenever I heard someone speaking German I couldn't help but wonder what their parents or grandparents might have done during the war. And on the rare occasions when I did visit this ancient homeland, I looked at every shopfront, every building, every person, wondering about their past during those terrible years.

Now I feel differently. I want to reclaim the citizenship that was stripped from my mother when she was seven years old because she always mourned the loss of her German home and I know she would have done the same if she were alive today. I want to draw a line under that past. With this small gesture of reconciliation I might be able to move on. It's not a question of forgiving, or forgetting. There are Jews who will be horrified by the numbers applying for dual citizenship of a country that could create the greatest catastrophe we have ever known, still a living memory for many. But as I come so much closer to my own death it feels important to show tolerance, to reach out and shake the hand of the one thing that has destroyed so much, just as I have had to do with cancer.

I will always cry when I see footage or hear testimony from those times, for their suffering, their horror, their trauma could have been my mother's, my grandparents', and it was the fate of my great-grandparents. But this is a different kind of gut feeling, a hope that by taking one active step I will find one small way to reclaim something that was stolen from us.

We visited the German embassy to apply for our passports on 8 June. Ironic timing. General Brexit Election day. After my morning stretch, oil and meditation I was about to throw on some jeans when I remembered how important it had been for my grandmother to always dress smartly. She wore sharp suits, silk shirts, fur stoles and elegant hats with intricate veils that would cover half of her face. A smart exterior could hide any amount of vulnerability. She was not and never would be considered a 'dirty Jew'. So I changed into something better – good trousers, heels and a black cashmere sweater so that I could also wear my mother's silver necklace from the sixties and take her to the embassy with us too on this auspicious day. When Nana died, my mother and I went through her jewellery together. Neither of us wanted much of it other than for sentimental reasons. Not to our taste but it did make me say to my mother, 'Well, there's only one thing I really want of yours: that scalloped silver necklace.' She had laughed. 'You can have that now,' she replied, going to her jewellery box to get it.

To become a German citizen you have to be there to accept the naturalisation certificate in person. We arrived early, went through intense security and were then showed to the office of Juliane, who had been processing our application. She explained how important the actual handing over of the certificate was, and then handed a piece of paper to me with the words 'I present to you, Catherine, your German citizenship.' I didn't think I would, but suddenly I began to cry. It makes me cry still just to write those words, for it felt like such a momentous step, after everything my family had been through. This wasn't just an insurance policy against Brexit, an escape hatch should things turn nasty here; this was a way of honouring my grandparents, great-grandparents and their suffering. Their names were already lodged in an archive somewhere in Germany, but now they are lodged in the embassy in London too: one more way of saying they are never forgotten. This was about righting a terrible wrong in a small but highly significant way – giving my family back the citizenship that was stolen from them. Our daughters and their children can apply for dual citizenship too as the German state tries to make amends for its past by welcoming back the whole family, which means even more to me. Who knows what sort of a future that will open up for them. But what I hadn't anticipated was what it felt like to accept that I am actually half German. The Nazis were my childhood monsters. They had produced the greatest genocide in history, in Europe, on our doorstep. By accepting German citizenship I can now finally acknowledge the positive aspects of that ancestry.

There was one final irony when we approached the passport desk. My brother had no trouble producing his fingerprints on the machine at the counter. Mine wouldn't take, however. The official kept asking me to wipe my fingers so that she could try again. I explained that I was on chemotherapy and that my fingerprints had been obliterated by the drugs, but she kept on wanting me to try and switched me to another machine on another counter. Still it wouldn't work. 'It won't affect your passport application – we'll just put a note in your file to say that the prints couldn't be taken. You could commit a crime!' she said.

I laughed. We have joked about that on several occasions. Only trouble is, they now use DNA.

My charming, charismatic oncologist is German and that helps with putting our history of persecution behind me too. I know that he is using his professional expertise to prolong my life when any one of his ancestors might have snatched it away. Somehow it feels important to trust him, even though I question the wisdom of taking oral chemotherapy daily, and ask him difficult questions whenever we meet. He doesn't know of my past, neither does my brilliant Chinese herbalist, who is also German. I wouldn't want to make either feel uncomfortable by telling them. But it feels so liberating to be able to reach out to others with a greater tolerance, just as new divisions and intolerances surface in Europe, driving some to suspect anyone different from themselves.

Getting cancer also means the end of living life in the middle lane, avoiding danger for a greater sense of (false) security. No more playing safe now. No more hiding from the world in case it should leap out and get me. No more worries about what things cost, or of losing everything. I can risk more now because I have less to lose and that's a very liberating thought. Too many days have been wasted in the past, time frittered away without stopping to notice beauty or create lasting memories with dear friends. But not any longer. There is no point in trying to avoid the depths of the darkest extremes of despair for they are already here, reminding me continually to rise up to the light of life and to live it. That's a gift, which only a fool would ignore, for in facing death I am finding so much more to live for than I ever thought possible.

Yesterday is gone and thinking about tomorrow is problematic, even upsetting. I make plans after good-news scans, when I am granted another few months of cancer-free life but looking any further ahead feels like arrogant wishful thinking. In some ways it is like turning back the clock and feeling really young again. The luxury of youth is that you cannot imagine a future where you might ever be old. You live only for the pleasures that come from the fresh experiences of each day – riding on the back of a boyfriend's motorbike at high speed without a helmet, hair flapping about in the warm wind; gate-crashing parties or running noisily through the streets with friends in the dead of night; smoking fat joints and drinking too much irrespective of what I might have to do with a hangover the following morning.

My life has been truncated. There is no length to it any more and it has all passed so quickly. Life is actually not much longer than a day, one glorious day. The sun comes up, throwing fresh light, making everything seem new and clean. Then it rises to full height and we bask in the illusion of constancy. This day is too good to ever end. But it begins to speed up and move more quickly towards the horizon and then slips quietly down behind the land and removes our limelight, our one short moment. Sunset throws out the same colours as autumn before the long dark night of winter.

Writing about the life that I have been lucky enough to have had allows me to live it again and to see that it has been full of vibrant activity, love and hope as well as times of despair. I have done a lot with these three score years. I just want another ten. Writing what will almost certainly be my last book feels like a full stop, bringing the work of thirty years to a close. For after new motherhood, adolescence, coupledom and infidelity, coping with mid-life and the close proximity of death has to be the last life stage. Not writing any more doesn't feel like a sad ending. I am not an author in search of another subject. I'm curious as to what else I might do to fill the void left in writing's wake. Accepting that things have come to an end isn't easy, but a space opens up just waiting to be filled with new activities, attitudes and love as well as a more open understanding and honesty about what really matters.

The clock is ticking for everyone; they just don't know it yet. The days and years are taken for granted until the prospect of future days and years are suddenly snatched away. Most can't hear time draining away like sand through an egg timer. But I can. And that's a privilege. With that knowledge embedded in every cell of my being, healthy and cancerous, I have no choice but to make the most of the life I have left. Clearly I would have preferred not to be this ill, or to have detected it sooner. But by always going to the good I can see that cancer has taught me something important – how love is all that matters, how important it is to show that love constantly to those I care about and build lasting memories which they can keep for as long as they live. Cancer has shown me how important it is just to get the best out of each and every day. I may have been suddenly thrown closer to death, but I have also, paradoxically, never felt more alive.

acknowledgements

I am so very lucky to have the best medical team – Prof Peter Schmid, Meena Sarin, Volker Scheid, Dr Helen Drew, Patricia Peat and Dr Wendy Denning. You are exceptional in your fields as well as being profoundly nice people. My respect, admiration and gratitude for everything that you do for me know no bounds.

Special thanks go to my agent Felicity Rubinstein and my publisher Lennie Goodings for so many years of good conversations about books and life, and for the great care they have given to all of my books. It has been a pleasure and an honour to work with you.

Thanks to Eleanor Wyld for the title and Orlando Weeks for the cover.

*

My love for Christoph, Eleanor, Grace, my family, my extended family and friends runs, I hope, like a very wide river through this book. If that hasn't been clear enough then here is one final word of farewell. It has been the greatest pleasure and honour of my life to love and to have been loved by you. And it is for all of you that I will do my damnedest to stay alive for as long as I can, even if all this anti-cancer activity takes up the best part of every day. For it is you that make my life worth living. Nothing matters to me more.